"Countless critters can thank Kristie for her incisive book and long-time advocacy of the Meatless Monday movement. Kristie combines personal stories, hard science, and practical suggestions that make going meatless easy and delicious on Monday . . . and any other day."

—Sid Lerner, chairman and founder, Meatless Monday

"I am convinced the single most powerful thing that any and all of us can do to make the world a better, kinder, and healthier place is incredibly simple and painless. Eat less meat (or none at all!). In her beautiful, thoughtful, and personal book, Kristie Middleton explains the how and why of that process and does so in a way that will surely change every reader's life in wonderfully positive ways. I highly recommend it!"

—Suzy Welch, bestselling author and TV commentator

"This work is perfectly timed. Just look at the *Journal of American Medical Association* from September 1, 2016. There is an analysis of the correlation of animal consumption and dying—relative to vegetable protein, all animal products produce cancer deaths, heart disease deaths, or both. Changing our entire health system from 'sickcare' to 'healthcare' is suddenly more critical than ever. One can imagine down the road that every patient who develops heart disease or cancer after a hospitalization would sue that institution and its staff for ignoring the peer-reviewed literature and bringing a food tray with our usual hospital food menu. Let's change it now. It's time to turn liability into opportunity!"

—Kim Allan Williams, Sr., MD, The James B. Herrick, MD, Professor of Heart Research; Chief, Division of Cardiology, Rush Medical College

"One of the most passionate leaders in animal welfare, Kristie creates an articulate plea for eating meatless—in defense of animals, people, and the planet. She follows this up with practical advice for how to make this happen in your own life, gleaned from her years of experience working with movers and shakers in the plant-based eating world."

—Sharon Palmer, RDN, the Plant-Powered Dietitian, author of *Plant-Powered for Life*

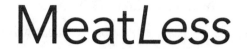

MeatLess

*Transform the Way You
Eat and Live—*
One Meal at a Time

Kristie Middleton

Da Capo
LIFE
LONG

Book production by Lori Hobkirk at the Book Factory
Designed by Cynthia Young
Set in 11.5 point Adobe Caslon Pro

Library of Congress Cataloging-in-Publication Data
Names: Middleton, Kristie, author.
Title: Meatless : transform the way you eat and live—
one meal at a time / by Kristie Middleton.
Description: Boston, MA : Da Capo Lifelong Books, [2017] | Includes index.
Identifiers: LCCN 2016043390 (print) | LCCN 2016046256 (ebook)
| ISBN 9780738219776 (hardcover) | ISBN 9780738219783 (ebook)
Subjects: LCSH: Vegetarianism. | Nutrition. | Animal welfare.
Classification: LCC TX392 .M53 2017 (print) | LCC TX392 (ebook) |
DDC 641.5/636—dc23
LC record available at https://lccn.loc.gov/2016043390

First Da Capo Press edition 2017
ISBN: 978-0-7382-1977-6 (hardcover)
ISBN: 978-0-7382-1978-3 (e-book)

Published by Da Capo Press, an imprint of Perseus Books, LLC,
a subsidiary of Hachette Book Group, Inc.
www.dacapopress.com

"Cage-Free, Free Range, Certified Humane: What Does It All Mean?" on page 22 is used with permission from the Humane Society of the United States.

Note: The information in this book is true and complete to the best of our knowledge. This book is intended only as an informative guide for those wishing to know more about health issues. In no way is this book intended to replace, countermand, or conflict with the advice given to you by your own physician. The ultimate decision concerning care should be made between you and your doctor. We strongly recommend you follow his or her advice. Information in this book is general and is offered with no guarantees on the part of the authors or Da Capo Press. The authors and publisher disclaim all liability in connection with the use of this book.

Da Capo Press books are available at special discounts for bulk purchases in the U.S. by corporations, institutions, and other organizations. For more information, please contact the Special Markets Department at the Perseus Books Group, 2300 Chestnut Street, Suite 200, Philadelphia, PA, 19103, or call (800) 810-4145, ext. 5000, or e-mail special.markets@perseusbooks.com.

10 9 8 7 6 5 4 3 2 1

To my animal companions past and present.

You've filled my life with unconditional love and inspiration.

And to the animals suffering on factory farms.

I see you, and I'm doing my best.

Contents

Introduction

I n December 2009, my husband, Mark, received an email from an animal sanctuary where he'd volunteered. The email requested that a group of us help transport several dozen "spent" egg-laying hens, who had been discarded by an egg factory farm, to the sanctuary. Mark explained that we'd leave early on a Saturday morning to meet the rescue agency, move the birds from their transport crates to comfortable boxes we'd prepare for them in advance, and then drive them a couple hours north. He asked if I'd like to come along but warned that I'd be seeing animals who had been through hell. I couldn't turn down the opportunity to help deliver these animals to a safe haven, but in spite of Mark's warnings, I wasn't fully prepared for what I would encounter.

When I saw these hens, I couldn't help but think of the time I was nine years old, and my older sister taunted me about the eggs I was eating:

"You know what that is, don't you?"

"What?" I asked.

"Dead baby birds."

As a nine-year-old, eggs happened to be the only food I knew how to cook. My uncle Rodney, who'd once stayed with my family for a month, taught me how to make scrambled eggs. To me, it was magic watching them go from liquid to congealed to cooked within moments of hitting the hot skillet. That was when I fell in love with cooking.

It took a moment for my sister's comment to hit me. *Dead baby birds*? I stopped eating eggs immediately.

Though I later learned that my sister was wrong—that the eggs we eat are actually unfertilized—as a child who loved animals, my sister's ribbing was sufficient to turn me off eggs for good. Twenty years later, during that rescue, I came face to face with the actual ugly truth behind the egg industry.

Having been involved in animal advocacy full time for many years, I knew that the majority of egg-laying hens are confined in wire mesh cages with up to seven other birds. I knew that virtually all of their natural behaviors are denied—dustbathing, perching, and even spreading their wings. But I was still shocked to see the condition of the birds.

On the cold winter day when we transported the hens, they arrived stuffed into tiny plastic crates with several other birds. Many were missing feathers, exposing raw, pink skin, and some had malformed beaks from botched debeaking (when factory farmers cut their beaks off with a hot blade to prevent them from pecking). They all had overgrown toenails from standing on wire for the last year or more, and some were too weak to stand up on their own.

Retirement for egg-laying hens typically means being gassed to death then sold as low-grade meat for pet food or farm animal feed. These fortunate birds would experience something much better. Upon arrival at the sanctuary, the hens were gently removed from the crates and placed inside a barn that had been prepared for them. At first they were tentative, but a few brave souls began exploring their surroundings. Watching the birds explore the solid ground under their claws instead of the cage wire to which they were accustomed was deeply moving. Some curiously scratched at the hay that had been placed on the ground while others pecked at it, and there were a few hens who were so weak they never stood up while we were there.

Slowly, the birds who had never properly exercised extended their wings, flapping them for the first time without touching the sides of their cages or one of their cage-mates. A few began taking dust baths, flinging the straw and dust up around them and relishing in the experience of cleaning their feathers. *This*, I thought, *is why I work every day to help animals.*

Caring about animals is something I've done from the time I was a young girl. Like most children, I had a natural affinity for animals and adored the animals I grew up with. As a small child growing up in Chesapeake, Virginia, I'd recite the following prayer nightly:

Now I lay me down to sleep,
I pray the Lord my soul to keep;
If I shall die before I wake,
I pray the Lord my soul to take.
Amen. God bless Mom, Dad, Jenny, Tinker, KC, Pete, Garfield, Elvira, Bud.

"Mom, Dad, and Jenny" are pretty obvious. And the others? The rest of the family: Tinker, KC, and Pete were our dogs; Garfield was my goldfish; Elvira was a parakeet; and little ol' Bud was a Siberian hamster. (If you think hamsters are cute, you haven't seen cute until you've seen one of these guys.)

I grew up in suburban America with a typical childhood: spending time outdoors playing with my friends, riding my bike, and vegging out watching cartoons on Saturday mornings and MTV after school. My pets were always at my side—they were family members whom I loved dearly.

My diet was also typical. I grew up eating Kraft macaroni and cheese, McDonald's hamburgers, and Chick-fil-A nuggets. At one point, in my early teens, I considered becoming vegetarian. I bought a container of water-packed tofu, drained the water, and tried eating the blob for dinner—plain, unadorned, and flavorless. And there ended my first experiment with vegetarian eating. (If I could share but one gem of wisdom, it'd be this: don't try eating plain tofu for dinner!)

Later in life, my college marketing professor discussed the concept of euphemisms—how words can make unpleasant things sound more appealing. She asked how appealing it would be to eat chicken nuggets if we instead called them "processed flesh of dead animals."

Her words affected me. I'd sit down to eat a sandwich and think about eating the "flesh of dead animals." I couldn't do it, so I became a vegetarian.

Around that time, I started volunteering for an animal protection organization and became aware of the myriad ways humans use animals—for food, research, entertainment, and more. So, I decided to work full time to help animals, and that's what I've been doing ever since.

Today, I'm senior director of food policy for the Humane Society of the United States (HSUS)—the nation's largest animal protection organization. In the nearly two decades I've been working in this field, I've seen tremendous progress: the number of animals euthanized in shelters has decreased dramatically, cruel farming practices once considered standard are now illegal in some places, and animal cruelty and dogfighting are now felonies in all fifty states.

These transformations are happening because, as a society, we care deeply about animals. From the time we're young, we're taught to have compassion for animals. We're exposed to animals throughout childhood in seemingly endless ways. Who didn't have a favorite stuffed animal as a kid? We watch animals on cartoons, wear animal print clothing, and read stories prominently featuring animals such as *Charlotte's Web* and *The Tale of Peter Rabbit*.

And we live with lots of animals. According to the American Pet Products Association, nearly 80 million US households—65 percent of us—have animal companions. Forty-two percent of those homes with animals have more than one.[1]

As it turns out, our animal affinity extends to those animals raised for food. Technomic, a foodservice industry research and consulting firm, found animal welfare to be the third most-important social issue to restaurant-goers.

Yet while we want animals to be treated humanely, there remains a cognitive dissonance in which our daily actions don't necessarily align with our values. According to 2015 polling by the Vegetarian Resource Group (VRG), only 3.4 percent of Americans are vegetarians—the same percentage of Americans who reported to be vegetarian in 2009.

However, VRG also found that 47 percent of us eat meat-free meals at least one day a week.[2] In fact, USDA figures indicate that we're eating 10 percent less meat now than in 2007. So though the number of us becoming vegetarian or vegan remains consistent, the number of us actively reducing the meat we eat is growing. As a society that loves animals, we haven't succeeded in reconciling our love of animals and how we eat. Yet that's beginning to change with more of us desiring to eat less meat—for animals, our health, or for the planet.

Transitioning to vegetarian was easy for me: I was exposed to information that I found compelling and made simple changes to what I ate; I continued cooking my favorite meals but made them without meat; I sampled new vegetarian products at health food stores and ventured to new restaurants to try food that was brand new to me.

Although I'd stopped eating shell eggs as a child, I still consumed them in baked goods. As a new vegan, I experimented with baking with egg replacers. I tasted a variety of dairy-free milks and swapped my cows' milk for soymilk. And I explored ice creams made from almonds and rice milk instead of dairy.

Although the shift from omnivore to vegetarian to vegan was a slow process for me, I have friends who became vegan overnight, and others who are enjoying more plant-based meals while still eating meat from time to time. Everyone is at a different place in their transition: maybe you're thinking of committing to a vegetarian or vegan lifestyle, or maybe you want to be more of a flexitarian and reduce the amount of meat you eat while still eating meat occasionally. Whatever path you choose, we can all eat healthier and more in alignment with our values.

Of course, eating more plant-based foods and less meat will be better for our health. Numerous studies conclude that overconsumption of meat is associated with obesity, and the most common preventable causes of death such as heart disease, cancer, and stroke.[3] On the other hand, eating a more plant-based diet has been found to help improve weight management and to prevent and even reverse these illnesses that claim millions of lives prematurely every year.[4]

Plant-based eating is also better for the environment and animals. To produce the large quantity of meat and other animal products we consume each year, the United States grows (and imports) vast quantities of grains, funneling them through billions of animals. That's an inefficient way of producing protein and causes land, water, and air pollution and creates greenhouse gas emissions.

And those billions of animals are often warehoused in cramped facilities, stuffed into cages and crates barely larger than their bodies—like those hens I helped rescue had been—and abused in ways that most people would find unacceptable.

Fortunately, the tide is turning toward a healthier future for all, with Americans' recent reduction in meat consumption and move to make vegetables the center of our plates. Eating more plant-based foods and less meat is becoming wildly popular. In 2015, a food industry publication, *Foodservice Director* magazine, named the most popular menu stories and "Vegan Went Mainstream" came in at the top.[5]

Sir Paul McCartney, Senator Cory Booker, Reverend Al Sharpton, Al Gore, Beyoncé, and Jay Z: every month it seems we hear of a new celebrity or public figure who's eating a meat-free diet to lose weight, stay fit, or help animals. How'd forty-five-year-old Jennifer Lopez drop 10 pounds? She went vegan, embracing what the *Daily Mail* called "Hollywood's hottest eating plan."[6]

It's not just Hollywood. As an employee of the HSUS, I work with institutions nationwide, helping them add more meatless options to their menus. More than two hundred K–12 school districts—including in Kansas City, Detroit, San Diego, Houston, and Los Angeles—are participating in programs like Meatless Monday. Hospital systems nationwide are reducing their meat usage. There are even some public schools and a county jail that have gone 100 percent vegetarian every day of the week.[7]

With more of us eating less meat, we've found ourselves at a crossroads. On one hand, we have big corporations tantalizing us with inhumane and unhealthy food products, and our waistlines continue to grow. On the other hand, we're desperate to take control of our health, we want to align the way we eat with our moral compass, and we've been taking steps to get there. We're searching high and low for easy answers, and companies desperate for a buck are feeding off our food frustrations: from plans to avoid carbs and pile bacon high on our plates to plans that would have us eat like cavemen—everyone is trying to sell a magic bullet.

Meat*Less* is about shedding the burden of the old model of dieting and sacrifice—it's about reclaiming our health, eating greener, and sparing animals. It's about exploring, cooking, and enjoying new foods. It's about turning away from the notion that we need a slab of meat at every meal and instead enjoying delicious, clean meals that are packed with all the vitamins, minerals, and nutrients we need—meals that will energize us rather than slow us down. We can each liberate our plates from always having meat at the center, just as millions are already doing.

Wherever you may be on this journey, this book will meet you there. My goal is to help explore why going meat*less* is a healthy choice—and one with so many other benefits—and to help you find your way. With simple strategies, recipes, swaps, ingredient talk, and more, together we'll find an approach that works for you. Get ready . . . we're going to make many changes.

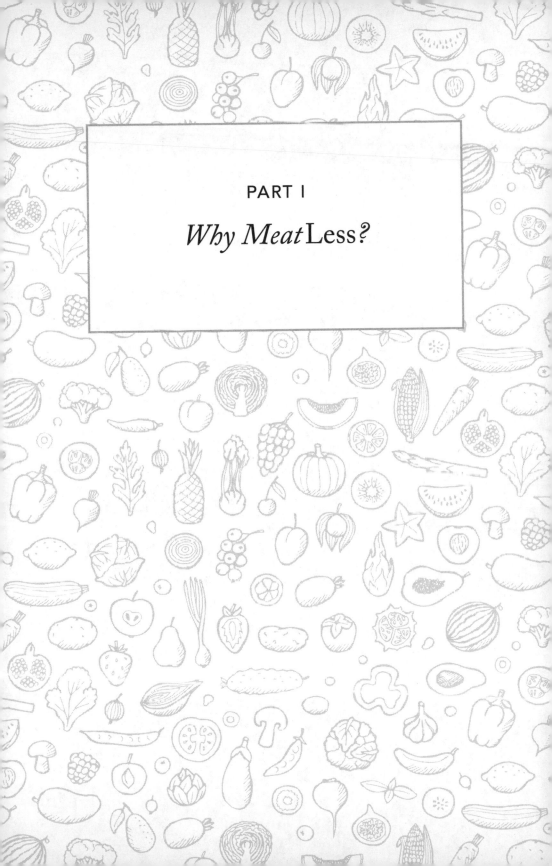

PART I

Why Meat Less?

1

Eating Ourselves to Death

Few people can say that watching television changed their life, but that's exactly what happened to Eric O'Grey. The Whirlpool Corporation area sales manager was watching CNN one evening when he saw former president Bill Clinton being interviewed by Wolf Blitzer about Clinton's new diet: plant-based and mostly vegan.

O'Grey watched the former commander in chief discuss his struggles with heart disease and fast food and the healing power of his newly adopted plant-based diet. The president looked great. He said he felt great. Inspired by the interview, O'Grey thought, *If Bill Clinton can transform his health and life, why can't I?*

Indeed, O'Grey's health needed transforming.

"In August 2010, I weighed 340 pounds and had type 2 diabetes," he confessed. "My waist size was 52. I couldn't fly on an airplane without a seat belt extension. My cholesterol was 300 and my blood pressure was stratospheric. I couldn't walk up stairs without getting winded. I was spending more than $1,000 each month for medications to treat high blood pressure, cholesterol, and diabetes. My doctor advised me to have weight reduction surgery and told me if I didn't reduce my weight, I might as well purchase a cemetery plot."[1]

O'Grey took immediate action. He purchased *The China Study*—a book about the link between chronic illnesses and animal product consumption. He sought help from a nutritionist, who taught him what to eat and how to cook using a variety of fruits, vegetables, and whole grains while avoiding meat, dairy, and eggs.

O'Grey had never consciously incorporated meat-free meals into his diet—the majority of his meals were acquired from delivery or drive-through. But he began replacing all animal products in his home with protein-packed plant foods such as quinoa, tofu, and beans. He added more fresh foods like kale, tomatoes, and mushrooms. He figured out which staples in his diet were already plant-based—cereal, bread, pasta, potatoes, and rice. And he implemented a moderate exercise program of walking his newly adopted dog, Peety, for thirty minutes each day.

And it worked: O'Grey lost more than 100 pounds in seven months. His weight dropped to 175 pounds, and his blood glucose levels returned to normal. His waist size decreased to 32 inches. His cholesterol dropped to 114. His blood pressure became normal. And he was able to stop taking medications. His newfound health allowed O'Grey to take up running and, in 2012, he ran seven full marathons and 15 half marathons—even qualifying for the Boston Marathon. Just a few years before, struggling to climb a single flight of stairs, O'Grey's new life would have seemed impossible.

Did you know?

More than one-third of US adults are obese. Part-time vegetarians weigh on average 15 pounds less than meat eaters.[3]

Five years after breaking free of animal products, O'Grey says his "energy, health, and weight continue to be optimal," adding, "I'm satisfied with my food, and have no food cravings or desire to overeat."

O'Grey, who made the adjustment to a plant-based diet with ease in just a few months, was most surprised that eating meat-free didn't mean giving up his favorite foods.

"My favorite dishes are what I call *vegan comfort foods*, such as lasagna, Mexican, Chinese, and similar international cuisines," he says. "So when people ask me what I eat, I turn the question around and ask them what they like to eat. When they answer my question, I explain how to make those same dishes without animal products."[2]

Plant-Strong for Life

O'Grey's inspirational story is just one of many from people who've changed their lives and revolutionized their health by adopting a plant-based diet. For some, the change comes easy; for others, change is hard. Consider the smoking physician or the overweight dietitian. We may know what's good for our health, but aligning our lifestyles accordingly doesn't always come easily.

Yet, most of us have some goals for change. We want to eat healthier, we want to quit smoking, and we want to focus more on the positive and less on the negative. It may seem hard, and sometimes impossible, but rest assured, it can be done.

We're living in an exciting time because so many people are taking the first step to make changes. Americans are embracing healthier eating—studies are showing we're consuming fewer calories and less meat—and it couldn't have come soon enough.[4] The Centers for Disease Control and Prevention (CDC) reports that the leading cause of death in the United States is heart disease.[5] It's likely many of us know someone who has suffered from this sad, often diet-related fate.[6] In fact, it's so prevalent that someone in the United States dies from heart disease every sixty seconds.

Many people tend to think of these conditions as inevitable or age-related; many resign themselves to taking medications in middle age to stave them off. But what if you were to learn that the leading causes of death weren't necessarily inevitable and, in fact, could be prevented with simple dietary changes? Would you make some simple changes to your diet and lifestyle if it meant you could live a longer life, look better, and feel fitter? Most of us would. And it turns out, we can.

To begin to solve this public health crisis, we must first look at its cause. Heart disease, according to the Mayo Clinic, "refers to conditions that involve narrowed or blocked blood vessels that can lead to a heart attack, chest pain (angina), or stroke."[7] When your blood vessels become narrowed or obstructed, it prevents your heart, brain, or other parts of your body from receiving enough blood. The University of Southern California's Keck Medical School simplifies it for us: "A non-clinical analogy would be a traffic jam on a highway."[8]

As Dr. Dean Ornish, the president and founder of the nonprofit Preventive Medicine Research Institute further explains, "Heart disease results when your heart becomes starved for oxygen that the blood carries. In part, this can be caused when blockages build up in the arteries that feed the heart."[9]

What causes plaque to build up, leading to blockages in the first place? According to W. C. Roberts, editor-in-chief of the *American Journal of Cardiology*, "It's the cholesterol, stupid!" (His words, not mine!)[10] Cholesterol is a waxy substance found in all of our body's cells. It's animal-derived, which means meat, eggs, and dairy all contain cholesterol.[11] And although we need cholesterol in order for our body to function properly, our body already produces all that we need.[12]

Yet we keep eating diets high in animal products. In fact, in the United States we eat more meat per capita than almost any other country in the world.[13]

The good news, though, is that we're learning more about the causes of these lifestyle illnesses, and some pioneering researchers are finding innovative solutions—and preventions—and people are listening and ready to make changes.

Dr. Caldwell Esselstyn and his peers at the Center for Lifestyle Medicine of the Wellness Institute of the Cleveland Clinic in Ohio found, "The epidemic of cardiovascular disease is nonexistent in cultures that thrive predominantly on whole foods, plant-based nutrition."[14] In an *Experimental & Clinical Cardiology* article, Dr. Esselstyn presents a powerful case for patients who suffered heart disease and later adopted a whole foods, plant-based diet. The patients who had previously undergone stents, tried prescription drugs, and after much frustration tried a plant-based diet found that the change in diet was what ultimately arrested and reversed their disease.

Losing Weight, Feeling Great

Nearly 80 million US adults—more than one-third of us—are obese.[15] Although we're no longer the most obese nation in the world (Mexico has taken the lead), let's face it: we're fat, and we're getting fatter. Dr. Eric Finkelstein with Duke University's Global Health Institute predicts that by 2030, up to 42 percent of Americans will be obese.[16]

This is more than just a cosmetic issue, of course. Conditions relating to obesity include heart disease, type 2 diabetes, some cancers, and stroke—many of the same conditions that top the list of the leading causes of death.[17] Dr. Michael Greger, a physician, bestselling author of *How Not to Die* and public health expert, combed through the world's nutrition research to put together NutritionFacts.org. Having looked at thousands of peer-reviewed journal articles on health and nutrition, he cleverly points out, "Death in America is largely a foodborne illness."[18]

> **Did you know?**
>
> Individuals who live in Blue Zones—five global regions with some of the longest-lived people in the world—eat primarily plant-based diets.[19]

Quite simply, there's an abundance of support for reducing meat, egg, and dairy intake in order to lose weight.

"A diet that promotes meat consumption might increase your risk of becoming obese," researchers concluded at the Johns Hopkins Bloomberg School of Public Health.[20] Dr. Youfa Wang and colleagues at Johns Hopkins reported findings of a consistent positive association between obesity and meat consumption.

Reducing the amount of meat we eat can help us with weight management.[21] People who eat meat-free tend to have a lower risk of obesity, according to the American Heart Association, because they typically eat less fat, including saturated fat and cholesterol, than those who eat meat.[22] In fact, in a study presented at the Obesity Society's 2013 annual conference, Dr. Brie Turner-McGrievy revealed results of the first randomized study that found "participants consuming vegan and vegetarian diets lost an average of 8.2 to 9.9 pounds over eight weeks, while those consuming some meat lost 5.1 pounds."

Okay, by now you might be thinking I'm trying to tell you that reducing meat consumption is a cure-all; I'm not. It won't solve all your problems. It won't make you rich. It won't ensure your children get straight As. But there's ample evidence that eating more plant-based food and less animal-based food is better for our health.

As it is, we're consuming foods that are laden with fat and cholesterol, and these foods may be cutting years off our lives. As doctors Greger, Esselstyn, McDougall, and so many others in this field show us, it doesn't have to be that way. We can live full, satisfying, and active lives well into our golden years. We can stay fit, look and feel great, and eat delicious, nourishing foods by making simple lifestyle changes.

You don't need to eat a 100 percent plant-based diet in order to make a difference. As healthcare providers at Kaiser Permanente tell patients in a guide to plant-based eating, "Any movement toward more plants and fewer animal products can improve your health."[23] In a nutritional update for doctors on this topic, Kaiser physicians write, "The benefits we realize will be relative to how many animal products we consume."[24]

Today, millions of Americans are eating with this recommendation in mind. Many are simply incorporating more plant-based foods into their diets. Others, like Eric O'Grey, are switching entirely to plant-based foods. The common thread among the many people reducing their meat consumption, regardless of the degree to which they make the change, is that they've chosen to live a healthier, happier lifestyle—starting with their plate. This choice is aligned with today's best science and is supported by some of the best minds in health and nutrition.

2

A Tale of Two Chickens

My parents live in rural Virginia on several acres of land they rent to a local soybean farmer. They have a small flock of chickens: a few hens and one rooster, Henry. They initially started keeping chickens after I brought them a few broiler chickens—what the industry calls chickens raised for meat—who had been rescued from a factory farm. They've had a few flocks over the years and enjoy them as companions because of their silly antics and the occasional egg they lay. The chickens live in a spacious run with two areas for pecking around for worms and bugs and investigating. Inside the safety of the henhouse, they have nesting boxes in which to lay their eggs and perches to stand on.

Sitting at the kitchen table during a recent visit, I watched Henry poke his head through the chain-link fence to reach a blade of grass outside the enclosure. I'd traveled to rural Virginia from my home in California to visit my family and to enjoy a change of scenery, and I empathized with Henry's desire for the same. I asked my father if we could let the birds out. "Sure. How you gonna get 'em back in?" he asked. I didn't wait to answer. My sister, niece, nephew, and I trekked outside to let the birds out to enjoy the day with us.

All but one of the chickens—Lyle, named after Lyle Lovett because of their similar "hairstyle"—tentatively crept out to explore. (My parents later discovered Lyle was a female when she started laying eggs, but the name stuck.) Quickly, they disappeared under the soybeans, which were at the height of their maturity, obscuring the birds completely. I instantly understood my father's question about corralling them back into their enclosure.

Henry was my saving grace. He stood on the side of the field and moved with the hens, monitoring their positions. While they were safely exploring, protected by the cover of the plants, he stood vulnerable to predators, doing his job monitoring their locations and looking for dangers. If they moved toward the back of the field, so did Henry. The girls and Henry were communicating all the while. The hens might make a little chortle when they found something good to eat. Henry would call out to check in, and they'd call back to reassure him. And when a hawk flew overhead, Henry delivered an alarm call to warn the girls, who were safely under the cover of the soybeans.

The hawk concerned me, though, as I certainly didn't want any part in putting the hens in jeopardy. My father, amused at being correct, pulled on his tall boots and waded into the field to flush the birds out. My nephew Liam, entertained by the whole business, asked why Henry wasn't following the hens into the field. Dad responded that Henry was doing his job to keep watch and protect the hens. Much to my relief, my father was able to lure the hens and Henry back into their run with relative ease.

I love my family dearly and always relish our time together, but I took only a few photos of them during that trip. Most of the pictures I took were of the chickens. It was incredible to see the differences in their personalities. Some are tentative and skittish while others are outgoing and inquisitive. There was shy Lyle, who never left the coop where the birds sleep at night, let alone the outdoor enclosure where they spend their days. And Henry, the fiercely protective rooster who stood guard and made sure his flock was safe. Watching the birds, I was reminded how every animal on this planet has a personality and is an individual.

The Chicken and the Egg

Although many of us are eating less meat to live longer, many are also doing it to avoid taking animals' lives. Indeed, in greater numbers than ever before, we're concerned with the toll our broken food system takes on animals. A 2007 poll commissioned by the American Farm Bureau Federation found that 95 percent of consumers say they want farm animals to be treated well. Yet the reality is that nearly every animal raised for food today languishes inside a crowded factory, rather than on a farm—a victim of inhumane agricultural practices.[1]

It's ironic because, let's face it, we are animal-loving people. The number of households with pets more than tripled between the 1970s and 2012.[2] We treat them like family, throwing them birthday parties, allowing them to sleep in bed with us, and mourning the loss of their lives as we would a human friend. We dress them in silly clothes and lavish them with gifts. In fact, the majority of us with pets buy them Christmas presents, with Americans spending $5 billion annually on holiday gifts for our animal companions.[3]

We do this because we love them. Because the animals with whom we share our lives and our homes make us laugh, comfort us when we feel alone, fascinate us with their personalities, and warm our hearts with their loyalty.

Animals raised for food share many similarities with the animals we consider our friends. I hadn't really spent much time around farm animals until my parents started raising chickens, but I quickly came to realize that although they look and sound (and smell!) different from the cats and dogs I was more familiar with, they also share many commonalities—such as how they communicate.

After spending some time with chickens, I realized their little warbles, squawks, and crows were more than mere noises. Chickens use at least twenty-four different cries to communicate with each other, including distinct alarm calls to warn one another of predators approaching by land and by air.[4] They form complex social structures—their pecking order. Although, to us, chickens might all look similar, they can recognize the facial features of more than one hundred other chickens.[5] If you look closely, you can see that every chicken has a unique face, just like every human has a unique face. And they feel for each other: scientists at the University of Bristol, in

England, found that chickens are capable of experiencing empathy, once thought to be a trait exclusive to human beings.[6]

Chickens are intelligent, too. Researchers in Italy proved that baby chicks are able to do basic math, adding and subtracting objects as researchers hid the objects behind screens.[7] (Maybe the next time we're called "birdbrained" we should take it as a compliment!)

One of the things I learned from watching my father's chickens was that they're extremely curious animals. They'll spend hours pecking around looking for seeds or bugs to eat or simply exploring their surroundings. This is the chicken version of our dogs sniffing to explore the neighborhood. They do it to learn about their surroundings and maybe find a treat or two along the way. And instead of showers, chickens take dust baths. They lie on the ground to cover their feathers in dust and then shake it off. *Why on earth do they do that?* You might wonder, as I did. It's their way of cleaning their feathers.[8] Think about your cat grooming herself by licking her body or her paw to clean behind her ears. Although we may not clean ourselves in the same way, we understand why they do it as they do.

Did you know?

Chickens have their own sophisticated language with at least twenty-four different sounds to communicate a variety of things like the threat of a predator or the exciting discovery of delicious food.[9]

At night, the chickens all made their way into the henhouse. As the sun went down, I watched them find spots on a perch, gripping the bar with their feet—a position in which they'd sleep until morning.

When we think of chickens, we tend to think of eggs. Wild chickens lay eggs primarily in the spring. When they're ready to lay, they leave the flock and find a secluded nest site in which to protect their brood, once hatched.[10] Domestic chickens retain this natural desire to have a safe, secluded nesting area to lay their eggs so that once their chicks are hatched they can watch over them safely. In fact, scientists have found that chickens care more about finding a secluded area to lay their eggs than about finding food after not eating for twenty-four hours.[11]

The term "mother hen," meaning a protective figure who fusses over others, exists for a reason.[12] Chicken mothers are extremely attentive to their young. They teach their chicks which foods are good to eat by calling to them and pecking at the ground. They also teach their young how to navigate their surroundings.[13] And they protect their young from predators by covering them under their outspread wings or by puffing up their feathers to lure predators to themselves and away from their chicks.[14] They want to protect their offspring like any mother would.

But chickens caught up in our industrial food system live in stark contrast to what chicken life is meant to be. Once birds who roamed the jungle floors while caring for their young and slept high up in trees at night to keep safe from predators, today's chickens are warehoused for life, the vast majority never seeing the light of day until they're packed into crates bound for the slaughterhouse.

Bad Eggs

On a hot July night in 2015, Isabelle Cnudde learned where eggs come from. As a volunteer with Animal Place, a Northern California sanctuary for farmed animals, Cnudde was on a team of volunteers who signed up to rescue hens from an egg factory farm that was disposing of its hens who were no longer laying a sufficient number of eggs.

The volunteers arrived at the farm at 1:30 a.m.—a deliberate decision to come at a time that would give them and the chickens they'd rescue relief from the oppressive summer heat and when the hens would be less active. It was pitch-dark as they approached the warehouse-sized buildings. Then it hit her: there was an overwhelming stench of ammonia, hanging so thick in the air it burned the volunteers' eyes as they worked. "As you approach the cages, you can see three to four feet of poop. There are a lot of critters living in the manure: cockroaches, flies of course," she recounted.

Cage-Free, Free Range, Certified Humane: What Does It All Mean?

A brief guide to what labels on meat and dairy products mean for animal welfare from the Humane Society of the United States website.

An abundance of labels on meat and dairy products make such claims as "grass fed," "cage-free" and "natural." What exactly do these labels mean, especially in terms of animal welfare?

Nearly all animal products in the United States come from factory farms. Some of the claims on product packaging represent better conditions for animals than those suffered by animals raised on factory farms, while others don't relate to the animals' welfare at all. So, how meaningful are these labels?

Here are the most common labels, decoded.[15]

CERTIFIED ORGANIC

The animals must be allowed outdoor access, with ruminants—cows, sheep, and goats—given access to pasture, but the amount, duration, and quality of outdoor access is undefined. Animals must be provided with bedding materials. Though the use of hormones and antibiotics is prohibited, painful surgical procedures without any pain relief are permitted. These are requirements under the National Organic Program regulations, and compliance is verified through third-party auditing.

Some labels mean that the animals have access to the outdoors, but there's often no regulation of the amount or quality of that access.

FREE-RANGE CHICKENS AND TURKEYS

The birds should have outdoor access. However, no information on stocking density, the frequency or duration of how much outdoor access must be provided, nor the quality of the land accessible to the animals is defined. Painful surgical procedures without any pain relief are permitted. Producers must submit affidavits to the US Department of Agriculture that support their animal production claims in order to receive approval for this label.

GRASS-FED

Ruminant animals are fed a diet solely comprised of grass and forage, with the exception of milk consumed before they are weaned. These animals have access to the outdoors and are able to engage in some natural behaviors, such as grazing. They must have continuous access to pasture during the growing season (defined as "the time period extending from the average date of the last frost in spring to the average date of the first frost in the fall in the local area of production"). Painful surgical procedures without any pain relief are permitted. Producers must submit affidavits to the USDA that support their animal production claims in order to receive approval for this label.

Global Animal Partnership 5-Step Animal Welfare Rating Program

Animals are raised according to different levels of welfare standards, from Step 1 to Step 5+. In essence, Step 1 prohibits cages and crates. Step 2 requires environmental enrichment for indoor production systems; Step 3, outdoor access; Step 4, pasture-based production; Step 5, an animal-centered approach with all physical alterations prohibited; and, finally, Step 5+, the entire life of the animal spent on the same integrated farm, with all transport disallowed. Hormone and subtherapeutic antibiotic use is prohibited. The 5-Step program is audited and certified by independent third-parties. The 5-Step Animal Welfare Rating Program is the initiative of Global Animal Partnership.

ANIMAL WELFARE APPROVED

The animals have access to the outdoors and are able to engage in natural behavior. No cages or crates may be used to confine the animals, and growth hormones and non-therapeutic antibiotics are disallowed. Some surgical mutilations, such as beak-mutilation of egg-laying hens, are prohibited, while others, such as castration without painkiller, are permitted. Compliance is verified through auditing by the labeling program. Animal Welfare Approved is a program of the Animal Welfare Institute.

CERTIFIED HUMANE

The animals must be kept in conditions that allow for exercise and freedom of movement. As such, crates, cages and tethers are prohibited. Outdoor

(Continues)

access is not required for poultry or pigs, but is required for other species. Stocking densities are specified to prevent the overcrowding of animals. All animals must be provided with bedding materials. Hormone and non-therapeutic antibiotic use is prohibited. Pain relief must be used for physical alterations (castration and disbudding) for cattle. For other mammals, anesthesia and analgesia must be used over seven days of age, but not earlier. Poultry may have parts of their beaks removed without painkiller, though not after ten days of age. The program also covers slaughter methods. Compliance is verified through auditing by the labeling program. Certified Humane is a program of Humane Farm Animal Care.

NO TAIL DOCKING

In the United States, some dairy cows have up to two-thirds of their tails amputated without anesthetic, usually by using tight rubber bands to restrict blood flow until the tail detaches, or is cut off with a sharp instrument. This is painful and renders the cows less able to fend off flies. Some dairy producers label their milk specifically as "no tail docking" to let consumers know their cows have full tails. There may be some verification of this claim, but not necessarily.

Labels like hormone-free don't carry significant relevance to the living conditions of the animals.

HORMONE-FREE, RBGH-FREE, RBST-FREE AND
NO HORMONES ADDED

These labels on dairy products mean the cows were not dosed with rBGH or rBST, genetically engineered hormones that increase milk production. Hormones are commonly used to speed growth in beef production, and their use by both the beef and dairy industries is associated with animal welfare problems. Chicken and pig producers are not legally allowed to use hormones. These claims do not have significant relevance to the animals' living conditions. There may be some verification of this claim, but not necessarily.

CAGE-FREE

Unlike birds raised for eggs, those raised for meat are rarely caged prior to transport for slaughter. As such, this label on poultry meat products has virtually no relevance to animal welfare. However, the label is helpful when found on egg cartons, as most egg-laying hens are kept in severely restrictive cages prohibiting most natural behavior, including spreading their wings.

VEGETARIAN-FED

These animals may be given a more natural feed than that received by most factory-farmed animals, but this claim does not have significant relevance to the animals' living conditions. As well, some farm animals, such as pigs and chickens, are not natural vegetarians anyway.

DOLPHIN-SAFE

In the United States, a Dolphin Safe label on a can of tuna means that no dolphins were intentionally chased, encircled, traumatized, injured, or killed in order to catch tuna swimming beneath the dolphins. Due to pressure from other countries, the US government has made multiple attempts to weaken the rules and allow the use of the label even if the tuna were caught by deliberately setting nets on dolphins. The HSUS and others have won a series of lawsuits to maintain the integrity of the label, so a Dolphin Safe label in the United States still means that the tuna were not caught using methods that harm dolphins.

NATURAL AND NATURALLY RAISED

These claims have no relevance to animal welfare.

GRAIN-FED

This claim has little relevance to animal welfare, but feeding ruminants—cows, sheep and goats—high levels of grain can cause liver abscesses and problems with lameness. As such, beef products labeled "grain-fed" most likely come from animals who suffered lower welfare than beef products labeled "grass-fed."

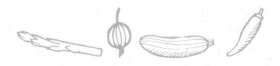

It wasn't the smell that bothered her most, though, but what she saw when they got close.

"The first thing I saw was white hens floating in midair like little ghosts in the shed," she said. "It looked surreal. Coming closer, I saw the cages were hanging from the ceiling with all the hens inside." Packed inside the shed were thousands of hens crammed into cages. The chickens inside were in pitiful shape. They had almost no feathers, especially around their necks, as they have to stretch their necks through the cage wires in order to reach the food.

They were debeaked—the ends of their beaks had been seared off, which is a common industry practice done to prevent the birds who are packed together so unnaturally tightly from pecking one another. Some of their beaks were mutilated so badly the birds had difficulty eating. Many had claws so long they couldn't put their feet flat on the ground. This was because of having never been able to scratch. In the end, the rescuers brought fifteen hundred hens to safety. There were some they couldn't save—they simply didn't have the space for them all.

"About seven hundred hens remained, and I knew they would be killed," she explained with a heavy voice. "I had to focus on the ones we saved."

Back at the sanctuary, Cnudde and the volunteers had the joy of watching these birds who had been caged their whole lives take their first steps. Some flew out of the cages, and some were shy.

"They poke their heads through and you may have to help them," she said. "What most of them do right away is start taking dust baths in the straw. They are full of lice. They've been itching for the last two years with no relief. All of them stretch their wings. Some of them try to fly. They scratch, jump, and flap. They've never been able to use their wings."

Cnudde brought two birds home. She named them Marjo and Tarra, and they enjoy spending their evenings pecking around the secure coop Cnudde and her husband built in their backyard. Their days are spent scratching around the yard looking for insects, sunbathing, taking dust baths, and enjoying their favorite foods such as tomatoes and kale. Although she'd love to see an end to all cage confinement, Cnudde knows at the very least that she's giving these hens the best possible lives she can. If only all chickens could experience the same.[16]

Overwhelmingly, the eggs on supermarket shelves come from factory farmed hens. The birds are confined with five to seven other birds in "battery" cages roughly the size of a desk drawer. Typically, each caged hen is afforded only 67 square inches of cage space—less space than an iPad—on which to live her entire life. The cages, stacked tier upon tier and row after row, may confine hundreds of thousands of birds in a single factory.

The things that chickens do in the wild and which are so important for their welfare—dust bathing, perching, and nesting, for example— are impossible to do in battery cages. In the absence of anything to peck in these cages, some hens, driven by boredom with their barren surroundings and their desire to explore their world with their beaks, will peck one another's feathers. Rather than addressing the extreme confinement and lack of environmental enrichments, the majority in the agribusiness industry instead debeaks them—all without painkillers, which had been done to the hens Cnudde and the other volunteers rescued.

"Virtually all aspects of hen behavior are thwarted" in these cages, wrote Dr. Bernard Rollin with the Department of Animal Science at Colorado State University in his book, *Farm Animal Welfare: Social, Bioethical, and Research Issues*. "Social behavior, nesting behavior, the ability to move and flap wings, dust bathing, space requirements, scratching for food, exercise, pecking at objects on the ground. . . . The most obvious problem is lack of exercise and natural movement. . . . Research has confirmed what common sense already knew—animals built to move must move."[17]

Broiler chickens—those raised for meat—don't fare much better. We farm them more than any other land animal, slaughtering more than 8.5 billion annually for human consumption in the United States alone—about 287 animals per second, every second of every day.[18]

These broilers are typically confined in large, warehouse-like "grow-out" sheds. The facilities are usually barren, save for litter on the floor and automatic feeders and waterers.

For chickens to reach market weight faster, the agribusiness industry has selectively bred broilers for rapid growth and massive size. In 1920, a chicken reached 2.2 pounds in sixteen weeks. In the early 2000s, a broiler may reach 5.9 pounds in only six weeks, at which point she'll be sent to slaughter.[19] According to researchers at the University of Arkansas, if human beings grew as fast as modern broilers, a 6.6-pound newborn would weigh 660 pounds in just two months.[20]

Because of this faster-than-natural growth, the birds are prone to crippling leg deformities, weak bones, and even heart failure when their organs can't keep up with the growth of the rest of their bodies.[21] Since they often grow so large their legs are unable to support their bodies, they spend their time lying in their own defecation.[22]

When the birds reach about six to seven weeks old, the birds who have survived are rounded up, grabbed by their legs, turned upside down, and carried, five or six at a time, by a worker, who then crams them into transport crates for the journey to the slaughterhouse.[23]

According to the Southern Poverty Law Center, "Speed is crucial to this line of work. Chicken catchers say they are paid a group rate for catching the birds . . . and there is no additional compensation for working more than forty hours a week. One chicken catcher said he typically worked with a crew of seven or eight workers who were required, at each henhouse they visited, to catch 24,000 or more chickens, usually within three hours. This means each worker had to catch and load about 1,000 chickens each hour, or about 17 chickens per minute."[24] Many birds suffer bruises, broken bones, and internal injuries in the process of being caught.[25]

Josh Balk, a former undercover investigator who works at the Humane Society of the United States, describes his experience working at a chicken slaughter plant: "At the slaughterhouse, the birds are snatched from their transport crates upon arrival, hung upside down, and thrust into shackles. Since speed is the objective, the animals' welfare is the last consideration. I saw birds that were picked up by their necks, legs, or wings and slammed into the shackles so hard I couldn't believe that their legs weren't ripped right off."[26]

Once shackled, a conveyor belt moves the hanging birds through an electrified water tank meant to immobilize them. Birds experience painful electric shocks, as their wings make contact with the water; others are able to lift their heads and miss the water entirely. They then move on to the next phase: the throat-cutter.

The birds are meant to die from blood loss after their throats are cut, after which they are dragged through a water scalding tank for defeathering. Balk witnessed birds who missed the automated blade because they were improperly shackled and therefore went into the tanks filled with scalding hot water while still fully conscious.

"The unfortunate birds that went into the scalding tanks while alive experienced an even more gruesome, agonizing death than those birds whose throats were slit," he said. "These animals were essentially drowned to death in boiling water so rife with the fecal matter of the birds who went before them, the industry has dubbed it 'fecal soup.' I will never forget the feeling of seeing the carcasses of these animals completely lifeless when just moments prior, each and every one was an individual; each and every one carried the spark of life, which was extinguished for our appetites."[27]

[Getting the] Pig Out

On a crisp November day in 2012, I found myself zipping up a jumpsuit in a locker room with a group of food industry representatives. Along with representatives from some of the world's biggest food companies, I'd taken an hour-long bus ride that morning from Philadelphia to the rural outpost of Kennett Square where the University of Pennsylvania's Swine Teaching and Research Center is housed. We were there to see alternative methods of housing for gestating pigs—pregnant pigs used to breed the babies who'd end up in the nation's food supply.

The pressure had been increasing on the food industry, which had come under fire for the use of gestation crates for mother pigs.

Outlawed in ten states and in the European Union because of their cruelty, gestation crates are small cages that confine mother pigs for the duration of their pregnancy, which lasts four months. They're put into another crate to give birth, and then they are artificially inseminated and put back into the gestation crate. This cycle continues for about four years, so it amounts to virtual immobilization for these sensitive animals for their entire lives.

Pigs are highly intelligent animals—some scientists say even smarter than dogs—and perform better on intelligence tests than some species of primates.

Dr. Thomas Parsons, professor of swine production medicine, our host for the visit at University of Pennsylvania, told us how the Electronic Sow Feeding (ESF) equipment worked in their alternative "group housing" facility. Each pig was fitted with an ear tag containing an electronic identification read by a computer. She enters a stall, the transponder identifies her, and her daily ration is released inside the ESF where she consumes her feed without interference from other pigs—one reason the industry gave for keeping them in the gestation crates—to reduce food aggression.

The savvy pigs at UPenn quickly learned that the ear tags were responsible for releasing the food rations and began stealing one another's ear tags! The researchers scrambled and learned they needed to insert a radio-frequency identification tag (RFID) into the pigs' ears to keep them from cheating.

Did you know?

In addition to being highly intelligent, pigs have complex emotional lives. Researchers have found that they can be optimistic or pessimistic because of their living conditions.[28]

Pigs are also very social animals, so confining them in these crates that prevent them from even turning around for their entire lives is very detrimental to both their physical and their psychological well-being. None of us would confine our beloved cat or dog in a tiny crate that prevents them from doing anything more than taking a step forward or backward for years on end, yet it happens every single day to mother pigs across the country.

Fortunately, the tide is turning on this inhumane practice. More than sixty of the world's largest companies such as McDonalds, Burger King, Safeway, Smithfield Foods—the world's largest pork supplier—and many, many more—some of those companies represented at our farm tour—have now committed to phasing out the use of gestation crates in their supply chain. And scientists like Dr. Temple Grandin, one of the foremost experts in farm animal care issues, are vehemently opposed to the use of gestation crates and are calling for their end. Dr. Grandin likened them to people living their entire lives in an airplane seat. Any of us who've been in the dreaded middle seat on a flight know it's pretty uncomfortable to spend five or six hours there. Imagine living like that for your entire life. It would most certainly be sheer torture.

Giving Thanks

The first time I ever met a turkey was at an animal sanctuary's Thanksgiving event. Harvest Home, a farmed animal sanctuary in Stockton, California, hosts an annual "Toast to the Turkeys" where it invites members of the public to meet animals that most people only encounter on their plates and enjoy a delicious meal while the animals also enjoy a Thanksgiving feast.

I encountered Kona the turkey in his enclosure where he was being admired by a young couple. He stood aplomb, slowly turning toward me to strut in my direction with his feathers puffed out and his tail feathers fanned. He was magnificent in his beauty but, I'd have to admit, a little intimidating. I quickly learned, though, that this gentle giant was quite the ladies' man. The feather puffing and fanning is courtship behavior. Kona wanted attention. I sat with him, fascinated for an hour, as he showcased his beauty to anyone who would give him some time, purring and periodically puffing his feathers and clearly enjoying the admiration of his visitors.

Kona, and all turkeys—both wild and domesticated—are fascinating animals. Having spotted them in my neighborhood in the

Oakland, California, hills, I've found that turkeys are majestic and inquisitive. That's not a new observation: Benjamin Franklin referred to them as "respectable" and even suggested we make the turkey our national bird.

Respectable indeed. Wild turkeys are adept communicators. They make at least thirty different calls to one another, including mating calls and calls to give specific warnings—such as whether they've encountered a rattlesnake rather than a grey rat snake, or if a hawk is flying overhead. They're also social animals, staying together in flocks.

These wild turkeys are fascinating individuals who share similarities with the millions of turkeys who end up on Americans' tables every Thanksgiving. They have similar social structures, vocalizations, and desires to protect their young.

Unlike their wild cousins though, nearly all commercially raised turkeys are raised on factory farms. These birds are packed wing-to-wing inside sheds the size of football fields—very different from their natural habitat. They're confined in this barren, ammonia-filled environment for the duration of their lives without any outdoor access.

Also concerning is that these birds have been genetically manipulated. The turkeys sold in supermarkets today look dramatically different from the birds our Native American and pilgrim forefathers—and even our grandparents—feasted on.

Through selective breeding, along with drug-laced feed, commercial turkeys have become Frankenfood. Today's factory-farmed turkeys grow far larger and faster than turkeys of the past. They have more than doubled in size from the Depression to today, ballooning from an average 13 pounds to an obese 29. They grow so large that not only can they not fly, but also they can't even mate on their own. That's right— the vast majority of turkeys ending up on holiday tables were bred using manual artificial insemination.

In the wild, these lithe, sleek birds are capable of running up to 25 miles per hour and flying up to 55 miles per hour. Due to selective breeding, factory-farmed turkeys are often unable to walk more than a few steps by the end of their brief lives. These turkeys may suffer crippling foot and leg deformities, and because they grow so large so fast, many suffer heart attacks, as their hearts aren't able to pump enough blood to support the rest of their overgrown bodies. If they don't succumb to fatal disease or injury, turkeys are typically sent to slaughter at around five months old.

Unfortunately, this is the tip of the iceberg. It's a lot to take in—and there's so much more to know about the way we treat animals. If you want to read more, visit humanesociety.org.

WHEN VISITING MY parents' chickens, I'm reminded that all of these animals these sensitive, inquisitive, interesting creatures—have likes and dislikes and individual preferences. They have lives worth living. They share with us, and the rest of the animal kingdom, so many basic desires—desires they are systematically deprived of when they are factory farmed by the millions. I see their freedom each time I'm at my parents' house, each time I watch Henry and the girls exploring their natural surroundings, and envision a future where all animals will be so fortunate.

3

It's Getting Hot in Here

Quiet and unassuming, Ben Peterson probably wouldn't come to mind when you think of an undercover factory farm investigator. Yet Peterson went undercover at a major turkey producer to document, and shine a spotlight on, how animals are often used and cruelly abused in agriculture.

Peterson worked the "live hang" and "re-hang" lines at a turkey slaughterhouse, where his shifts were spent pulling turkeys from their cages in the transport trucks on which they arrived and hanging them upside down in shackles by their legs. Later, after the birds were killed, he rehung the 40-pound carcasses.

"I started on the live hang line, and after just one day I got really sick. I couldn't keep food in me. I went to urgent care as soon as I could. I ended up losing 15 pounds in two weeks," the already slender Peterson recounted. "It's a tough job. It's nonstop repetitive, heavy lifting."[1]

The conditions were difficult. Workers were able to take short breaks—a few minutes, at most—from the intense labor and the extreme heat.

"It's so hot, it was hard to keep the respirator mask on," said Peterson. "And the animals are so freaked out that they're clawing and scratching and flapping all over the place. By the end of the day, you're covered in turkey shit."

Slaughter lines move quickly to process the eighteen thousand animals the meat industry slaughters every single minute of every day.

Very soon after starting the job, Peterson developed repetitive motion injuries. Within just one week of working on the live hang line, his arms would seize up and his fingers would curl uncontrollably.

Disregard for the animals' well-being was expected by management in favor of speed and efficiency. One day, Peterson found a turkey whose legs had been caught in the cage. He worked to gently remove him and was reproached by a supervisor who told him, "You have to yank the fucker out of there."

According to Peterson, on another occasion there was a bird who arrived unable to stand. A worker kicked the injured animal from the highest level of the unloading dock into the pit, a fall of about 15 feet. The bird was later run over and killed by the next truck to enter the dock. All of this happened in front of a US Department of Agriculture inspector who neither said nor did anything about it.

Peterson experienced psychological trauma, as many working in this industry do.

"After doing it for a while, at night, as soon as I started to fall asleep, I'd be back on the line with turkeys hanging in front of me," he recounted, tears welling up in his eyes.

> **Did you know?**
>
> Meatpacking has been consistently ranked as one of the most dangerous jobs in America. Illness and injuries in the meat industry are two and a half times the national average.[2]

The turnover was ridiculously high because of the difficult working conditions. More than half the people who started working at the same time as Peterson were gone by the end of his two months there. When he told his supervisor he was leaving to go back to school, Peterson was told to do it while he could, that he wouldn't want to work there for the rest of his life.

Peterson's experience is common among meat industry workers: grueling, physical work amid frenzied, frightened animals, causing injuries and psychological trauma.

The people who work in factory farm settings and slaughterhouses are paid low wages, typically have little-to-no experience working with animals, are given minimal training, and work in poor conditions. A 2015 Oxfam exposé on conditions for poultry processing workers revealed harsh, dangerous conditions.

"Roughly 250,000 poultry workers earn poverty level wages with few benefits; suffer injuries and illnesses at high rates, and then may be prevented from receiving proper medical care; and work in a climate of fear where they are afraid to speak out about the injustices they suffer," according to the organization.[3] Perhaps one of the most shocking findings is that workers at some of the nation's largest poultry producers are routinely denied bathroom breaks and thus deliberately dehydrate themselves, wear diapers to work, or urinate or defecate on themselves while working on the line.[4]

Josh Balk, the undercover investigator from Chapter 2 who worked at a chicken slaughterhouse, recalls watching several hours of training videos during his first day on the job, yet not a single video discussed proper treatment of animals, nor did anyone ever mention animal welfare.

Whether working inside the factory farms, catching chickens to cram them into slaughterhouse-bound crates, or working slaughterhouse lines, animal agriculture is dirty, difficult work. As Peterson saw firsthand, the US Government Accountability Office (GAO) reports that young male Latino workers represent the largest number of workers in the meat industry, which has one of the highest rates of illness of any US industry.

"They work in hazardous conditions involving loud noise, sharp tools, and dangerous machinery," the GAO writes. "Many workers must stand for long periods of time wielding knives and hooks to slaughter or process meat on a production line that moves very quickly. Workers responsible for cleaning the plant must use strong chemicals and hot pressurized water."[5]

Like Peterson, workers often endure a range of injuries, including burns, cuts, and repetitive stress disorders. Due to the dangerous nature of the job, serious injuries, such as amputation, fractures, and fatalities also occur.[6] Workers are routinely exposed to toxic chemicals, blood, and fecal matter, leading to illnesses.[7] Officials from Occupational Safety and Health Administration (OSHA) acknowledge that slowing down the production line could help reduce workers' injuries, yet the animal agriculture industry opposes even this modest reform.

As a result of the lack of training and difficult working conditions, animals are often victimized by employees who are desensitized by their work. Undercover investigations have documented extreme acts of sadistic cruelty, such as cows being punched in the face by workers and jabbed with electric prods, turkeys being kicked as though they're footballs and stomped on, and piglets being grabbed by their tender ears and thrown across the room.[8] This is how much of our meat travels to our plate. There's no question our industrialized food system is broken.

Healing Our Planet: Reducing Animal Agriculture's Impact

To buy a house and some land, to raise a family—it's the American dream. It was the dream of eighty-four-year-old widow Lita Galicinao and her beloved husband, Sam. They met in the Philippines during World War II, when he liberated her hometown. After the war, Sam brought his "GI Bride" back to the United States to fulfill their dreams. During the early 1950s, with several other families, Sam and Lita pooled their money and purchased 72 acres of land in Lathrop, California.[9]

Lathrop is in San Joaquin County, in California's Central Valley, 70 miles east of San Francisco. Peaceful and sunny, the Central Valley is one of the world's most productive agricultural regions.

Unfortunately, as agriculture moved away from family farming and toward industrialization, the American dream for Galicinao and her neighbors became more like a nightmare. In the 1990s, a nearby egg factory farm switched ownership. The new owners, Olivera Egg Ranch, expanded the facility to house up to 700,000 birds. Although its name may conjure pastoral images of birds foraging on a lush ranch, the reality for these birds was anything but: they were all confined in cages. Trapping hundreds of thousands of birds in cages is both detrimental to their welfare and presents additional problems, such as what do to with their waste. Olivera's solution was to dump the 133,000 pounds of manure generated daily into massive cesspools where it sat untreated.[10]

Those cesspools produced ammonia fumes so strong, Galicinao and her neighbors suffered for years, complaining of nausea, burning eyes, trouble breathing, and chest pains.[11] Plus, the putrid stench attracted flies that invaded neighbors' homes, further degrading their quality of life.[12]

In 2011, in response to a lawsuit filed against the egg factory by the Humane Society of the United States, a judge ordered Olivera to pay half a million dollars in damages to neighbors who lived closest to the cesspool.[13] Some may say this was a victory for Galicinao and the other residents who had suffered for decades because of the factory farm's negligence. Yet we're all losing because the system is still broken: the very means in which this factory farm disposed of its waste is common in the animal agriculture industry.

Did you know?

A hamburger requires fourteen times more water to produce than a veggie burger.[15]

The story of Galicinao and her neighbors is just the tip of the iceberg—factory farming's impact on the planet extends far beyond local cesspools.

With the expectation that we'll be feeding 8 billion humans by 2025, concern is mounting about the long-term sustainability of our meat-centric diets.

The 2010 study *Forecasting Potential Global Environmental Costs of Livestock Production 2000–2050* states, "As the human species runs the final course of rapid population growth before beginning to level off midcentury, and food systems expand at commensurate pace, reining in the global livestock sector should be considered a key leverage point for averting irreversible ecological change and moving humanity toward a safe and sustainable operating space."[14]

We are speeding blindly down a dead-end road, and we need to act fast to start putting on the brakes.

Water Wars

When Donna Johnson turned on the faucet in her Porterville, California, kitchen in the spring of 2014, a trickle of water came out and then nothing at all.[16] Johnson and her husband, Howard, live in Tulare County in the parched Central Valley. The county is in one of the regions of the state hardest hit by the four-year-long drought California began to experience beginning in 2012, prompting Governor Jerry Brown to declare a state of emergency.

Howard tried to extend the well—the family's source of water—to no avail. He should've tapped into a splash of water, but what he encountered instead was a hapless thud.[17] They started talking to neighbors and soon realized they were one family of hundreds in the community without running water.

As of April 2015, the county had recorded 996 well failures like those of Howard and Donna.[18] For her part, Donna, who became known locally as the "water angel," began delivering bottled water to her neighbors who were without running water. The county intervened as well, installing public showers and doling out bottled water.[19] The lack of running water makes life immensely difficult for these residents, affecting how they live and how they eat. Even the most mundane, everyday tasks such as cooking, doing dishes, and doing laundry become massive undertakings without water.

The situation for the Johnsons (and their neighbors who were also without water) may be extreme, but during the drought millions of Californians were required to undergo water restrictions, which were lifted by Governor Brown in the spring of 2016. Californians ripped out their lawns and replaced them with drought-tolerant plants, took shorter showers, and some of them "let it mellow." In spite of the restrictions being lifted, California residents were not out of the woods in 2016. The California Department of Water Resources said in April 2016, "The state's historic drought is far from over" and encouraged residents to "make the sparing, wise use of water a daily habit."[20]

What many people don't realize, though, is we could do far more to reduce our overall water usage by retooling what's on our plates than by reducing household water use, because animal agriculture is one of the biggest water users. In fact, research from the Pacific Institute implicates animal feed as being the single largest water user in California.[21]

Animal products have a significant water footprint. In fact, researchers found that it takes about one hundred times more water to produce 1 kilogram of animal protein than to produce 1 kilogram of grain protein.[22] Meat production is so water intensive that for the United Nations' World Water Day celebration, the agency's number one recommendation to participants is to "replace meat with another source of protein."[23]

Indeed, the average total amount of water needed to produce 1 pound of beef is 1,799 gallons, and 1 pound of pork is 576 gallons. The Monday Campaigns proclaims that for every burger we skip, we can save sufficient water to shower for two and a half months.

> **Did you know?**
>
> According to the Environmental Protection Agency about 1,100 gallons of water are needed to produce 2 pounds of chicken—not even an entire chicken (or a very tiny one). "That's enough water to fill about twenty-five bathtubs!"[24]

And it takes a whopping 880 gallons of water to produce just 1 gallon of cows' milk. By comparison, the amount of water needed to produce 1 pound of soybeans is 216 gallons, and the water needed for 1 gallon of soymilk is 49.4 gallons.[25]

Researchers Ercina, Aldaya, and Hoekstra, the world's foremost experts on water footprints of food, concluded, "The water footprint of the soy milk product analyzed in this study is 28 percent of the water footprint of the global average cow milk. The water footprint of the soy burger . . . is 7 percent of the water footprint of the average beef burger in the world."[26]

The majority of the water required to produce these foods is in the form of animal feed—primarily the water used to grow feed crops, accounting for 98 percent of the water footprint.[27] At least 80 percent of beef cattle in the United States are conventionally raised, meaning they consume grass in pasture, for their first twelve to fourteen months, and then are sent to a feedlot for three to six months to fatten them up prior to slaughter.[28] There, they eat a diet of soy and corn to speed up their growth—about 800 pounds of feed in the 140 days they spend at the feedlot.[29] It takes about 109 gallons of water to produce 1 pound of corn.[30]

California produces one-fifth of the nation's dairy milk, leading the nation in the production of dairy and butter, and it is second only to Wisconsin in cheese production.[31] As a spokesperson from the Tulare County Farm Bureau told the *Los Angeles Times*, "The average dairy here is 1,800 cows. . . . So a large-scale dairy farmer needs 126,000 gallons of water per day just for cows."[32]

Perhaps if we all reduced the amount of meat, eggs, and dairy we consume, Donna, Howard, and their Tulare County neighbors could turn the taps back on.

Something Stinks: Waste Intensity of Factory Farms

As the neighbors of Olivera Egg Ranch learned, confining hundreds of thousands of animals together in a concentrated area presents a waste disposal conundrum. Factory farms produce massive amounts of manure, in many instances generating as much waste as an entire city. The difference is that a city's municipal waste is treated, while manure from factory farms is dumped into giant lagoons or cesspools and then sprayed directly onto fields.[33]

Manure can be good for soil and has been a valuable fertilizer for centuries; but the amount of manure produced by factory farms is so vast that the soil can't absorb it.[34] The lagoons themselves emit toxic gases such as ammonia, hydrogen sulfide, and methane. Sometimes they leak, break, or in the event of a flood, may overflow, sending dangerous pollutants into water supplies.

North Carolinians witnessed this firsthand. In the fall of 2016, Hurricane Matthew deluged the state with torrential rain, causing massive flooding of the Tar, Neuse, and Lumber rivers. These precious waterways sit near hog and chicken factory farms, some of which were flooded during the storm. "The carcasses of several thousand drowned hogs and several million drowned chickens and turkeys were left behind," reported an article in the *Washington Post*. "An incalculable amount of animal waste was carried toward the ocean. Along the way, it could be contaminating the groundwater for the many people who rely on wells in this part of the state, as well as threatening the delicate ecosystems of tidal estuaries and bays."[35]

This was a near repeat of 1999's Hurricane Floyd, which ravaged the eastern part of the state. During Floyd, several manure lagoons ruptured and dozens flooded, spewing out millions of gallons of untreated waste and saturating already-oversaturated fields even more.[36]

More than 2 million turkeys, chickens, and pigs confined in factory farms were killed in the storm—many drowning to death.[37] The spilled manure, along with the decomposing corpses of tens of thousands of pigs, clogged coastal waterways and flowed into the Pamlico Sound—the nation's second-largest estuary and an important ecosystem for salt water–dependent wildlife. The waste resulted in a 350-square-mile "dead zone," an oxygen-deprived area of the ocean that kills all oxygen-dependent ocean life.[38] Waste from factory farms has contributed to a number of these major environmental disasters.

Energy Hog

Dr. Helen Harwatt has long been interested in protecting our natural environment. As a young college student, she was intrigued by geology and the natural world and ended up studying environmental sciences.

How Factory Farm Operations Pollute Waterways

- In 2015, a pipe burst on an Iowa pig factory farm, causing manure pits to overflow and spill into a nearby creek. This triggered a massive fish kill, the third reported that week.[39]

- In 2015, the Gulf of Mexico experienced one of the largest dead zones on record, stretching more than 6,400 square miles—about the area of Rhode Island and Connecticut combined—in which no sea life was able to survive.[40] Runoff from fertilizer used to grow animal feed is one of the most significant contributors to the dead zone, while manure from factory farms contributes an estimated 15 percent of the nitrogen flowing into the Gulf.[41]

- In 2014, the Chesapeake Bay, the nation's largest estuary, experienced a massive dead zone of more than 1 cubic mile.[42] Scientists attribute the dead zone to waste and runoff from nearby chicken farms. In 2014 alone, Maryland produced 280 million chickens—48 chickens for every resident in the state.[43]

- In 2014, manure from a Missouri hog farm spilled while it was being applied to fields, polluting a local tributary with ten thousand gallons of untreated pig waste.[44]

- In 2014, inspectors with the Central Valley Regional Water Board cited a California dairy for leaving "abundant cow bones in various stages of decay within large piles of manure solids" and for evidence "the lagoon had overflowed into adjacent cropland."[45]

- In 2014, half a million Ohio residents lost access to drinking water due to phosphorus runoff from farms and cattle feedlots, causing massive algal blooms in Lake Erie, some of which were poisonous.[46]

- In 2014, a North Carolina pig factory farm spilled 100,000 gallons of manure from a waste lagoon.[47]

- In 2014, a storm water system failed at a Michigan dairy, resulting in its manure lagoon spilling into nearby waterways at least five miles from the site.[49]

- In 2013, a Wisconsin dairy farm was fined $65,000 for polluting nearby groundwater with manure.[48]

- In 2013, a concrete wall of a manure pit fractured, spilling 1 million gallons of manure into two streams before making its way into a Minnesota river.[50]

- In 2012, a North Carolina dairy "failed to check and maintain the levels of cow waste in its on-site waste containment lagoons," resulting "in the spillover and discharge of 11,000 gallons of cow feces and other waste into the French Broad River."[51]

- In 2011, an Illinois hog farm overflowed, spilling 200,000 gallons of manure into a creek over a 19-mile stretch and killing more than 110,000 fish in the process.[52]

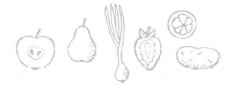

During her studies she gained a strong insight and appreciation for how intricately and delicately balanced the natural world is—and how much human interference threatens this balance. While studying at the University of Leeds in England, Harwatt became interested in climate change. It was the early 2000s, and climate change was a relatively new issue, yet some of her professors were discussing it. Fascinated, Harwatt became interested in behavior change and ways individuals can have an impact on reducing climate change. She completed her Ph.D. on transportation policy and climate change mitigation, looking at how driving our cars less can have an impact.

Harwatt soon learned, though, that what we eat plays an even bigger role in our impact on climate change than how we get from point A to point B. She became deeply frustrated to find that so few people were researching it, but a passion was ignited, leading Harwatt to move from Leeds in England all the way to Loma Linda University in Southern California where she serves as a research fellow and environmental nutritionist. There, she and her team study the impacts of our diets on human health and planetary health.

One of Harwatt's most surprising findings was the large extent to which animal foods contribute to our most serious and pressing environmental problems, including climate change, biodiversity loss, water pollution, and deforestation. The scale of production and the inefficiency involved in producing animal foods are largely to blame. Her colleague at Loma Linda University, Dr. Joan Sabaté, explains that there's a vast difference comparing the energy input and output of the production of meat versus that of plant protein. "Plant foods are eleven times more efficient than animal foods," he stated.

"The main issues relating to the inefficiency of animal agriculture relate to feed conversion, so calories in versus calories out," Harwatt explained, citing research from Gidon Eshel, professor of environmental science and physics at Bard College in New York.[53]

A study from the *American Journal of Clinical Nutrition* found that animals farmed in the United States consume more than seven times the amount of grain than the *entire American population* consumes directly.[54] Further, the researchers found that less cropland is used to

Table 3.1 Energy Required to Produce Animal Foods

PRODUCT	CALORIES OF PLANTS REQUIRED TO CONSUME 1 CALORIE
Beef	37
Pork	12
Chicken	9
Eggs	6
Dairy	6

Source: Wolfram Alpha Computational Knowledge Engine
Helen Harwatt, Ph.D.

produce food for a plant-based diet than a meat-based diet (less than 0.4 hectare of cropland compared to 0.5 hectare of cropland), as well as less fossil fuels, and less water.

Animal production is energy intensive, requiring fossil fuels to produce electricity for equipment and machinery and to run the factory farms themselves. Petroleum-based chemicals and fertilizers are used to produce crops that will be fed to animals.

Research published by The Royal Society, the United Kingdom's national academy of science, found, "The energies used per tonne of the main outputs of animal production are all substantially higher than crops. This results from the concentration effect, as animals are fed on crops and concentrate these into high-quality protein and other nutrients. Feed is the dominant term in energy use (average of about 75 percent), whether as concentrates, conserved forage, or grazed grass. Direct energy use includes managing extensive stock, space heating for young birds and piglets, and ventilation for pigs and poultry."[55]

"It seems ludicrous that we're using all these precious natural resources in such an inefficient way," Harwatt lamented. "It'd be much more efficient if we just grew plants instead of animals. The animal products are so inefficient. There's so much loss along the way." Simply put: producing meat requires more water, land, and energy than producing plant proteins.

Less Meat, Less Heat

Perhaps factory farming's greatest disaster is the role it plays in climate change. I recall, as a child, receiving mailings from environmental organizations, urging me to help "Save the Planet." I splayed the stickers across my notebooks and wrote papers about reducing greenhouse gas emissions. I diligently turned out the lights when I left a room, helped my parents recycle, hung our clothes out on the clothesline instead of using the dryer, and was mindful of my water use. We heard about a hole in the ozone layer and were warned to stay away from products containing chlorofluorocarbons (CFCs). Out went the aerosol hairspray—this in the big hair days of the 1980s. Little did I know then that what I put on my plate had a much bigger impact on reducing greenhouse gas emissions than swapping my hairspray for an inferior pump and all those other actions combined.

Abundant scientific evidence confirms that greenhouse gas emissions contribute to climate change—the greatest threat to human health in the twenty-first century, according to the World Health Organization, and perhaps the biggest threat to public health the world has ever known.[56] Increasingly, people are also becoming aware that meat, egg, and dairy production are major greenhouse gas emitters. The United Nations Food and Agriculture Organization estimated that animal agriculture is responsible for at least 14.5 percent of all human-induced greenhouse gas emissions.[57]

The US Environmental Protection Agency identified carbon dioxide (CO_2), methane (CH_4), nitrous oxide (N_2O), and fluorinated gases as the most significant greenhouse gases, with carbon dioxide representing 81 percent of US emissions, methane 11 percent, and nitrous oxide 6 percent.[58] These gases trap heat in the atmosphere—hence the name "greenhouse gases"—which are leading to the warming up of our planet.[59]

The Intergovernmental Panel on Climate Change states livestock are some of the largest global sources of methane and nitrous oxide—two particularly potent greenhouse gases—accounting for about one-third of global, human-induced emissions of methane.[60] A December

2014 report from think tank Chatham House suggests, as do other reports, that the livestock sector is a bigger contributor of greenhouse gas emissions than direct emissions from the entire transportation sector.[61]

According to the Environmental Defense Fund, "If every American skipped one meal of chicken per week and substituted vegetables and grains . . . the carbon dioxide savings would be the same as taking more than half a million cars off U.S. roads."

Animal agribusiness emits carbon dioxide—which is less potent than methane and nitrous oxide—primarily in the form of fossil fuels used to power equipment and farm machinery and to transport and store foods.[62] Methane is produced when ruminant animals (cows, goats, and sheep) digest food. Nitrous oxide is released into the atmosphere through animal manure as well as during the production of synthetic fertilizer, which is used on crops grown to feed animals. Chatham House states that animal agribusiness is also a large contributor to deforestation and the carbon dioxide (CO_2) emissions associated with deforestation, be it indirectly with the growing demand for animal feed crops expanding into forests and grasslands, and directly as forests are clear cut to create grazing areas and feed pastures.[63]

While attending the 2015 United Nations Conference of the Parties 21 (COP21) in Paris at which I participated in a panel discussion, I sat rapt in the audience as I listened to Roni Neff, Ph.D., assistant professor from The Johns Hopkins Center for a Livable Future. Neff shared a report that reviewed scientific literature on the role reducing food waste and animal product consumption plays in meeting climate change mitigation goals. World leaders from more than 150 countries converged to discuss ways to meet the agreed upon goal of preventing the planet's temperatures from rising an additional 2 degrees Celsius. Although Neff's organization is the scientific partner to the Meatless Monday campaign, its findings indicated that one meat-free day would be a good starting point, but even that wouldn't be enough to reach the target.

"Studies suggest that substantial global reductions in meat intake by 2050 could reduce agriculture-related emissions on the order of 55 to 72 percent, with greater reductions from also reducing dairy and eggs." Their research concluded we'd need a 31 percent reduction in global animal product intake, and regions with higher intake of animal products would have to reduce even more. Moving toward a diet with less meat, though, "represents an important first step toward the necessary dietary changes, particularly if adopting modest reductions in meat intake subsequently leads to greater dietary shifts."[64] One thing is certain: if we want to curb climate change, we must reduce our global meat, egg, and dairy consumption.[65]

A Chickpea in Every Pot

Concern is mounting that, given meat production's resource intensity, it's critical that we continue reducing our meat consumption if we're going to be able to feed the world. Microsoft cofounder and philanthropist Bill Gates has weighed in on this issue.

"By 2030, the world will need millions of tonnes more meat than it does today," wrote Gates. "But meeting that demand with animal products isn't sustainable. The meat market is ripe for reinvention."[66]

Ripe for reinvention and, indeed, in need of it. The amount of crops currently fed to farm animals could feed an extra 4 billion people.[67] International relief organization Oxfam estimates 795 million people suffer from chronic malnutrition worldwide.[68] That's right: We're feeding more grains to farm animals than would be needed to address global malnutrition. The United States alone expends 67 percent of its total calories on livestock feed. We could feed nearly three times as many people as we currently do by providing those calories from crops to humans rather than feeding them to animals. "The US agricultural system alone could feed 1 billion additional people by shifting crop calories to direct human consumption," wrote researchers from the University of Minnesota in the journal *Environmental Research Letters*.[69]

As for Helen Harwatt, when asked whether we should be concerned about food security, she said, "Based on what I've read in the scientific literature, I'm not concerned because I know that right now, we have the resources to feed that many people if we focus on plants." We're just not currently expending those resources in the most efficient way. Her recommendation for those interested in doing as much as they can to be a part of the solution is to strive for a whole foods, plant-based diet incorporating as much vegan and organic produce as possible. A small step, though, would be to replace meat with legumes, which she calls low-impact plant foods that can provide all the calories and protein we need.[70]

Fishing for a Solution

Okay, so we're feeding all these cows and pigs and chickens and turkeys all this grain, which is depriving the world of protein-rich plant foods, causing environmental disasters and generating animal suffering on a massive scale. But what about fish? Some people will say they don't eat land animals, but they do eat fish; is that any better? In a word: no.

There are health concerns regarding eating fish, including exposure to mercury and polychlorinated biphenyl (PCB), which are both toxins. Additionally, the methods in which fish are farmed, or wild caught, cause severe environmental damage.

Did you know?

Salmon contains nearly as much cholesterol as chicken (63 mg in 3-½ ounces versus 85 mg in 3-½ ounces, respectively). By comparison, ½ cup of pinto beans doesn't contain a single milligram of cholesterol, nor does ½ cup of tofu.[71]

Net Loss: How the Fishing Industry Is Impacting Our Oceans

Most of the fish consumed in the United States is still wild-caught. According to Marine Conservation Institute, "Today more than 25 percent of US fish stocks are overfished, which has led to the collapse of some very important fisheries and fishing communities."[72] The primary problem is the high demand for sea animals, and the methods used to catch those animals are problematic.

Trawling, for example, involves catching hundreds of thousands of pounds of sea animals in oceans worldwide. The fishing industry drags huge nets—about 150 feet wide (as wide as the Statue of Liberty is tall) and weighed down with heavy objects—along the ocean floor, netting up everything in their paths.[73] In addition to the fish intended to be caught, the trawlers often catch non-target animals, as well as corals, sponges, and other delicate and important ocean life.[74] Sea turtles, for example, which may live to be one hundred years old, may be caught. These animals must surface every twenty to thirty minutes for air, but when caught in trawling nets, unable to surface, they drown. The National Oceanic and Atmospheric Administration (NOAA) also implicates trawling as being responsible for turtles suffering broken shells or appendages, injuries, stress, and exhaustion.[75]

The great mammals of our oceans are also fishing industry victims. According to the Natural Resources Defense Council, fishing practices annually kill or injure nearly 750,000 marine mammals, including whales and dolphins.[76] With commercial whaling globally killing roughly 2,000 animals, clearly the greatest threat to whales isn't whaling boats, but rather our consumption of fish.[77]

For good reason, destructive fishing methods such as trawling are under fire from marine conservation organizations and consumers looking to embrace less harmful practices. If matters couldn't be worse in our oceans, overfishing is leading to the collapse of fish populations. *National Geographic* cites a study published in 2006 in the journal

Science, which predicts that if we continue fishing at current rates, "all the world's fisheries will have collapsed by the year 2048."[78]

As well, the decimation of ocean predators—of which about 90 percent have been destroyed—has resulted in unchecked populations of herbivorous ocean life, which are decimating coastal vegetation, a key source of carbon and thus a very important asset in climate change mitigation.[79] There truly is a circle of life.

Farmed and Dangerous

Now, fish farming has skyrocketed in the United States, making fish the second-most commonly farmed animal next to chickens, according to the Humane Society of the United States, with approximately 1.3 billion fish being farmed in aquaculture systems each year for food.[80]

Aquaculture typically involves confining fish in large tanks (closed systems) or at sea in open ocean farms enclosed by nets. The United Nations Food and Agriculture Organization reports that aquaculture accounts for nearly half of the world's fish.[81]

Like trawling, there are also severe problems with aquaculture, both open ocean and closed systems. Overcrowding is a threat for both types of aquaculture, which creates stress and spreads disease. In closed systems, this can also lead to water quality issues, making the animals susceptible to infections and other illnesses. In open ocean systems, wild fish and the surrounding environment may be threatened as well since there are no barriers to prevent the spread of disease, waste, or parasites.[82]

Something Feels Fishy

In addition to the impacts on our oceans, fishing—whether through trawling or aquaculture—also creates a moral dilemma. Fish are sentient and have unique personalities. The Panel on Animal Health and Welfare of the European Food Safety Authority wrote, "There is scientific evidence to support the assumption that some fish species have brain structures potentially capable of experiencing pain and fear."[83]

They can also experience pleasure. Journalist and hobby scuba diver Cathy Unruh shared the story of Larry, a grouper she encountered while scuba diving. "Whenever we would descend to his reef in the Bahamas, Larry would fishtail it over to us to engage in long, soulful eyelocks, slurp at our regulators, and get petted. He would roll from side to side and front to back to make sure we scratched every accessible scale."[84]

And surprising to many, fish are intelligent. Scientists at St. Andrews University found that nine-spined stickleback fish can observe others to make better choices, a trait not witnessed in other species.[85] Some fish have been observed using tools—using a rock to crush open the shells of bivalves (oysters, clams, and mussels)—which scientists consider to be very sophisticated behavior.[86]

Fish can even be caring parents to their young. Yet, we farm or catch them by the billions and then slaughter them in inhumane ways, such as simply letting them suffocate to death, cutting their gills with no stunning, or "live chilling" them, in which they're immersed in cold water.[87]

If all of that wasn't bad enough, according to Compassion in World Farming, "Many farmed fish are fed largely on wild fish. To produce farmed fish such as salmon, it takes about three times the weight of wild caught fish. This is not only unsustainable but adds to the serious welfare concerns about how wild fish are caught and slaughtered."[88] When we eat farmed fish, we're not just taking one life; we're taking the lives of all the fish killed to feed that fish.

Given the inefficiency and wastefulness of feeding wild fish to other fish, the environmental devastation of wild-catching fish, and the inhumane rearing and slaughter of farmed fish, it's no wonder that after looking at fish in an aquarium, novelist Franz Kafka is reported to have said, "Now I can look at you in peace; I don't eat you anymore."[89]

PART II

Getting Started

4

Aligning Our Plates with Our Values

So how do we get there? How can we free ourselves from fried chicken and break away from bacon? We know that eating too much of these products is bad for us, our planet, and animals. But there's no one-size-fits-all answer. Some people decide they want to go vegan and do so cold turkey (pun intended), while others opt for smaller changes such as going meat free one day a week. What works for one person may not necessarily work for you, and ultimately the best choice is always the one you stick with.

I was vegetarian for several years before learning about the benefits of a vegan diet and making that transition. Through the process, I learned about new foods that I'd never before tried. I ate sushi for the first time and learned you can order avocado, carrot, and cucumber rolls. Indian food was brand new to me. I explored Ethiopian, Thai, Vietnamese fare, and more—all foods I'd never eaten but loved immediately.

The journey turned out to be a wonderful one—if for no other reason because it so greatly expanded my culinary horizons. I now take pictures of my meals (yes, I'm that annoying person at the table), enjoy scouring through cookbooks for inspiration, and my weekend isn't complete without ambling through the farmers' market, taking in all the colors and sampling the delicious produce.

My transition was a slow one, as it often is for many others—eliminating chicken from their diet, then beef, then pork, and then dairy and eggs. Although some people have a lightbulb moment after watching a documentary or reading a book and immediately clear their freezers and refrigerators of animal products, others are simply enjoying more plant-based meals while still eating meat from time to time. As the saying goes, different strokes for different folks. The key is finding what's right for you.

The Incredible Shrinking Man

Argentina native Ken Chadwick, now the food service director for American University (AU) in Washington, DC, exudes passion for food. When speaking with Chadwick, his love for exquisite cuisine is clear. The great-grandson of Chilean cattle ranchers, Chadwick spent the summers of his youth herding cattle, and he spent his formative years living in major cities throughout South and Central America, informing his refined palate.

His passion for his job is clear too. Working as a food service director at a university setting often means long hours and juggling lots of responsibilities such as responding when things go wrong—when staff call in sick, when equipment breaks, or guests complain. And guests do complain. It can often be a thankless job. It can be a rewarding one too.

In September 2014, as he was starting his first year of operating the food services program at AU, Chadwick brought vegetarian and vegan students together to provide feedback on the campus dining options. Having worked at some of the most prestigious universities in the nation's capital such as Georgetown, Catholic University, and George Washington University, Chadwick was used to meeting the varied needs of his guests. He heard from many students at AU they wanted more vegan options, and at this meeting students said there simply still weren't enough. They were putting meatless options on the menus that he'd tested, but as he recounts, "The students had very reasonable complaints. Here was a staunch meat eater creating a vegetarian menu. My best wasn't even close."

As someone who is always motivated to do the best job possible, Chadwick was inspired. He wanted to see things from the students' perspective. He ended the meeting and declared that, as of the next day, he would be vegan. An all-or-nothing guy, he doesn't take a sip from the faucet; he, in his own words, "drinks from the firehose."

Very quickly Chadwick learned that it wasn't as easy as he thought to eat vegan on campus. With a laugh he shared, "The first day was a six-pear day. The first week was an all-pear week." He rallied the support of his dietitian Jo-Ann Jolly and that of chefs Norbert Roesch and Kyle Johnson to come up with unique options that would ensure that whether he was eating breakfast, lunch, or dinner on campus—and sometimes this workaholic dines on campus for all three—there was something vegan, hearty, and delicious he could enjoy.

Students at AU soon found options such as a falafel bar on campus where they can build their own wraps, roasted seasonal vegetables, marinated portobello mushroom caps, smashed English peas on toast, and so much more.

The menus weren't all that changed. Chadwick also found his own health improving. For years he'd been medicated for high cholesterol and high blood pressure. He was also overweight, his 6-foot-5 frame tipping the scales at 327 pounds. He had gastrointestinal issues and had to have his appendix and gall bladder removed in his late thirties.

"I was experiencing bone pain," he said. "I looked a million years old, and I wasn't happy."

When his gall bladder started acting up, the doctor marveled at the fact he was still alive. Chadwick was so overweight his doctor was worried he might die on the operating table, but his gall bladder was 97 percent non-functional, so they had no choice but to remove it.

His doctor warned him he should consider changing his diet, to which he replied, "Doc, it's not a meal unless it has meat in it." When Chadwick was at his heaviest, even getting dressed in the morning was a struggle. He recalls one painful memory of a morning when he was so overweight he couldn't lift his leg up high enough to put on his socks because of the girth of his stomach.

"I was sitting on the bed and had to lean on the side to pick my leg up and shimmy the sock on," he recounts. His then wife told him, "Baby, you're getting winded just putting your sock on," reminding him he was once a world-class athlete, playing football, basketball, and soccer, swimming, boxing, and doing martial arts. It was embarrassing and hurtful for anyone to see him like that.

So Chadwick started exercising. He'd struggle to finish a one-mile walk and would be in horrible pain all day. His knees hurt. But he was determined to lose weight, so he started running. He recalls running his first mile, and although he wasn't anywhere near home when he finished, he had to lie down in the grass and rest for an hour. After a while he was running five to six days a week, trying to remain at 320 pounds and not gain weight.

"It was a constant battle to remain at 320 pounds back then," he said.

So in the fall of 2014, when Chadwick dove in head first with his vegan diet, he found that the weight started dropping effortlessly. He lost 45 pounds by Christmas, shocking his family during the holidays. It happened so fast that his colleagues on campus dubbed him, "The Incredible Shrinking Man."

By the spring semester, Chadwick's weight was down to 250 pounds. Within six months, he was able to eliminate his blood pressure and cholesterol medication. Two years later, he told me with great enthusiasm, "I am down to 205 pounds! I haven't been this skinny since high school. Last Saturday I spent two and a half hours boxing then ran six miles, which I can do without even getting winded."

Chadwick added that he eats what he wants whenever he wants it. He never passes up food out of concern for his weight. He eats more consciously, though, and truly appreciates the foods he's eating.

"I want to understand where my food comes from, how it's handled, how it's being treated," he says. "The days of just slamming stuff into my mouth are gone."

Although he still eats vegan on campus and the majority of the time at home, there are some favorite foods that he eats on occasion. Oysters and softshell crabs, he confesses, are his weakness. They're available in the summer for a couple of months, so he might eat them once in a while when in season, or a piece of cheese here and there.

The vast majority of his meals, though, are plant-based. When asked what he eats, he shares a simple red lentil pasta recipe and describes the curries, chutneys, and dals that adorn his plate and appease his palate.

At forty-three, he's in much better shape than he was at thirty. He regrets that so many of his younger years were spent in abject pain because he hadn't connected how he ate to his health, which seems so obvious now.

"I'm a different person in so many ways," he said. Though he can't get those years back, he's grateful for the knowledge he's gained—and is passing it on. "I truly believe I'm one of the people making this worldwide change. I'm feeding 1,800 of some of the most influential, affluent kids in the nation at this institution every day in hopes one day they'll be in power and some of the things I've taught will make an impact."

Chadwick's advice to those who want to understand his experience? "It's nowhere near as hard as you think it is. It's far more enjoyable than you think it is. If I tell you the benefits, you won't believe me, so try it so you can see for yourself."[1]

The Psychology of Change

As Chadwick would attest from his attempts to lose weight, change can be hard. We're raised hearing that we need to exercise our willpower to do the things we should do and avoid doing the things we shouldn't. *Where there's a will, there's a way*, after all.

Yet as it turns out, it's not quite that simple. Psychologists have determined that willpower is an exhaustible resource that depletes throughout the day. Case Western Reserve University's department of psychology conducted some famous experiments to probe just how much power there is in our willpower.[2] Psychologist Dr. Roy Baumeister and his team had participants enter a room in which chocolate chip cookies had just been baked. In the room, fragrant with the smell of delicious cookies, was a table with a plate of said warm, fresh-baked cookies and a bowl of red and white radishes at which participants were seated. Some of the subjects were asked to eat the cookies while others were asked to eat the radishes. (Imagine sitting at a table smelling the aroma of freshly baked cookies and being asked to instead enjoy a raw radish or two!) The researchers left the room and returned shortly thereafter to present a puzzle for the participants to perform. They were given thirty minutes to complete a problem-solving task—a frustrating geometric puzzle.

Those participants who were told to eat the radishes and flex their willpower to resist the urge to eat the cookies gave up on the puzzle after about eight and a half minutes; those who were indulged with cookies continued trying to solve the puzzle for more than double the amount of time as their radish-eating counterparts!

The lesson here is not to eat cookies to give you the fortitude to complete a difficult task, as much as that does sound like a delicious idea. The conclusion the researchers drew was that the willpower required for participants to resist the cookies drained their self-control. "Wanting chocolate but eating radishes instead, especially under circumstances in which it would seemingly be easy and safe to snitch some chocolates, seems to have consumed some resource and therefore left people less able to persist at the puzzles," the researchers wrote.[3]

Several studies have concluded the same thing: willpower can be depleted. This may happen after a long day of hard work that involves making decisions. It may happen after exerting self-control and putting on a happy face around difficult people. And it may happen when we're trying to eat healthy foods over less-than-healthy foods. All of these situations are stressors on our self-control, and all of these situations exhaust our willpower. As Dan Heath, co-author of *Switch: How to Change Things When Change Is Hard*, writes, "Here's why this matters for change: In almost all change situations, you're substituting new, unfamiliar behaviors for old, comfortable ones, and that burns self-control."

If only that was all. Another barrier to change is our emotional mind versus our rational mind. Author Dr. Jonathan Haidt, who wrote *The Happiness Hypothesis*, famously described our rational mind as a rider atop an elephant and our emotional mind as the elephant.[4]

"I'm holding the reins in my hands, and by pulling one way or the other I can tell the elephant to turn, to stop, or to go," writes Haidt. "I can direct things, but only when the elephant doesn't have desires of his own. When the elephant really wants to do something, I'm no match for him."[5] We may have good intentions, and we may make decisions based on logic, but sometimes our elephant, our emotions, overpowers us. Sometimes we make decisions with our hearts (or stomachs!) instead of our heads.

So consider that next time you're confronted with choosing that familiar spaghetti with meatballs over the colorful pasta primavera. Your rider is going to direct you to the healthier vegetable-centric dish. Your elephant may go along with your rider, but sometimes he'll have a mind of his own. Sometimes your elephant will want the meatballs and will drag his heels; he may even rampage to get his way.

Indeed, we are not always in control of ourselves. We're creatures of habit, often finding a niche and sticking with it. Organ donation programs provide a great example. Psychologists Eric Johnson and Dan Goldstein compared the consent rates of organ donations in European countries. Germany uses an opt-in system, similar to the United States, in which citizens must give consent to be organ donors. There, 12 percent of the population consents to be donors. In Austria, on the other hand, officials use an opt-out program in which the population must refuse to donate. There, nearly the whole population, 99 percent of Austrians, donates their organs.[6] In another study, researchers found that when employees of a large corporation had to opt out of their company's 401(k) savings program (rather than actively electing to participate), participation was dramatically higher.[7]

What do either of these things have to do with how we eat? Newton's first law of motion states that an object at rest stays at rest, and an object in motion stays in motion. And you probably know from your own life and habits that there's a sort of behavioral inertia: simply put, we tend to stick with what we're doing because it's easier. But once we get started, once we make this new way our path, it will be easier for us to stay along the path. We just have to take the first steps. But how do we take those first steps?

How Do We Make Meat*Less* a Reality

So we have a limited amount of willpower, an unwieldy animal moving us along our path, an abundance of decisions to make, a real distaste for making decisions, and a tendency to stick to the easy, familiar route. No wonder change is difficult! Rather than fighting with our elephants and draining our willpower, why not work with them? We can use some simple, yet effective tricks to help making change become a smidgen easier.

Easy Strategies for Making Change Stick

Dr. Milena Esherick, program director at the Wright Institute graduate school of psychology in Berkeley, California, recommends using the following strategies (adapted from *Switch* by Chip and Dan Heath) for motivating oneself to make a successful shift to a plant-strong diet.[8]

Direct Your Rational Mind

- **Provide direction and few options**. Don't think about the big picture ("eat healthy"); think in terms of specific behaviors ("buy soymilk" or "try Meatless Monday").

- **Notice success**. When do you already eat plant-based foods? Do more of this. Replicate.

- **Point to the destination**. What is your goal? And why is it worth it?

Motivate Your Impulsive Mind

- **Build hope.** Knowledge isn't enough to change behavior; hope and belief in the ability to change facilitate actual change. The number-one predictor of our ability to be successful making any behavioral change is our belief that we can do it. When you've accomplished the goals you've set, no matter how low the bar is, celebrate those successes. When we realize we can be successful in the little changes we're making, we feel hopeful and are more motivated to make bigger changes.

- **Shrink change** so it's not overwhelming. Replace chicken nuggets with chicken-free nuggets, eat meatless on the weekends. Pick a regular meal (weekday breakfast, for example) to go meat*less*.

- **Make change part of your identity**. We make many decisions based on our identity. Ask yourself, *What would someone like me (an animal lover, a vegetarian, an environmentalist) eat in this situation?*

Shape the Path

- **Change your environment** to support a plant-strong diet. Make it easy to eat plant foods (fruit bowl on the counter, ready-to-eat meat-free snacks at eye level in the refrigerator, large serving dishes for meatless meals), and make it difficult to eat animal products (keep food out of sight and out of reach—wrapped in foil, high up in a cabinet, or in the garage).

- **Cue new habits**. Use cues in the environment to trigger new behavior. For example, if you're serving vegetables, make that a cue to serve yourself 20 percent more. If you go out to eat at a burrito joint, your habit can be to always order a burrito with rice, beans, and vegetables. Habits aren't always bad—in fact sometimes they can help us eliminate poor choices we'd otherwise make.

- **Rally the herd**. Eating habits are contagious. Help plant-based diets spread. (Eat plant-strong with others.)

Beyond Dr. Esherick's recommendations, there are more tips we can keep in mind to help us overcome the barriers to making change:

Make Your Intentions Clear. First, make clear, well-defined, realistic goals for yourself. Rather than, "I'm going to eat less meat," try "I'm going to eat vegetarian meals when I'm at home." Rather than, "I want to eat more plant-based meals," try "I will buy only meat- and dairy-free foods at the grocery store." Having these specific parameters will help present clarity as we're making our transition to eating more healthfully and humanely.

Share With Friends. Next, share your goal with someone—a friend or a spouse—or at least write it down. Did you know that verbalizing or writing down your goals can help you stick to them? According to psychology professor Gail Matthews at Dominican University in California, individuals who write down their goals will be 42 percent more likely to achieve them.[10]

To that end, enlist a friend to join you. Our eating habits are hugely influenced by our community. In research published in *The New England Journal of Medicine*, researchers found that an individual's likelihood of becoming obese rises by 37 percent if their spouse is obese, 40 percent if a sibling is, and 57 percent if a close friend is.[11] Dr. Walter Willett, chair of the department of nutrition at Harvard School of Public Health and co-author of *Thinfluence*, said, "Obesity is 'contagious,' but physical activity and healthy eating are too, so we want to emphasize the latter."

> **Did you know?**
>
> If we write down our goals, we're 42 percent more likely to achieve them.[9]

So if obesity is infectious, healthy habits can be too. Researchers have found that when we have a buddy to work out with, we're more likely to stick to our fitness goals and lose weight. In one study, subjects with at least one regular workout partner lost significantly more weight than those subjects who didn't have either a successful partner or who had no partner at all.[12]

If you're flying solo, try to find a community that will support your goals. There are Meetup groups everywhere in the country that could help support you (and you'll support others, too): from vegetarian animal lovers to vegan hikers to Meatless Monday potlucks and dine-outs—you can likely find a group (check out meetup.com, for example!) that would help introduce you to others moving on the same path.

Break Down Barriers and Set Yourself Up for Success. What about those other barriers, though—the depleting willpower that we rely on so much? Instead of fighting through difficult decisions, we can be more successful if we set ourselves up for success in advance. Simply planning ahead can make a difference. Think about the days you've packed your lunch the night before versus days when you rush out the door and have to grab lunch on the fly. Your lunches are likely a lot healthier (and cheaper!) when you pack them at home. Carving out time to do just that—packing lunches, creating a list of menus for what to eat during the week—will help tremendously.

Decide to Be the Decider. We tend to dislike making decisions, especially when there are many of them. To make that easier, we can create our own set of rules. For example, deciding that when we're cooking dinner at home we'll cook only meatless meals.

Creating shopping lists will help too. You've probably been warned not to go grocery shopping on an empty stomach; it's good advice. A study published in the journal *Health Psychology* had a group of dieters write down their weight-loss goals and the level of confidence that they'd achieve those goals. They also had them indicate how hungry they were. The dieters who were satiated had greater intentions for weight loss and more confidence that they'd meet those goals than did those dieters who were hungry, even mildly so.[13] So don't go to the grocery store hungry, and go with a shopping list and stick to it. Make it easier for yourself. If you know that you have a weakness for chicken nuggets, avoid that aisle unless there's something on your list you really have to have.

Embrace the Easy. Of course buying healthy food doesn't guarantee we're going to eat it. How can we ensure we make it easy to reach for a healthy, plant-based snack instead of an unhealthy one? Believe it or not, just seeing food may result in our eating more of it. Researchers tested this theory in which they gave office workers containers of chocolate kisses. Some containers were placed on top of the workers' desks, some were placed in a desk drawer, within reach but hidden from eyesight, and some were placed on a nearby shelf that would require the workers to leave their desks to reach the kisses.

What did they find? The office workers who had the candy on their desks visible throughout the day consumed 2.9 more candies on average than those workers who had the candies in a desk drawer. They ate 5.6 more candies than those whose candies were on a shelf that required they walk 6 feet to reach them. The researchers concluded, "We eat more of a food when it is 'in sight and in reach.'"[14]

We need to take convenience into account when making diet changes: make it inconvenient to eat foods we're trying to avoid and make it easy to eat foods we're trying to eat more of. Putting your fruit in a bowl on your counter immediately after purchase will increase the likelihood you'll eat it. We're less likely to grab a carrot to munch on throughout the day if we have to wash and peel it first. So wash and cut them and put them at eye level in the fridge—in a clear container, so they're the first thing you see when you reach in for a snack. When I was growing up, my mother knew I loved grapes, but they'd shrivel up and rot if she put them in the refrigerator in the bag in which they came. Simply by washing them, removing their stems, and putting them in a bowl, she'd ensure they'd be gone within twenty-four hours.

Change Your Environment. If a bowl of ice cream is your obstacle to eating more plant-based foods, consider changing your food environment. You can make it easier for yourself by simply not bringing the foods into your house that you want to avoid eating. I love sweets, and if they're in the cupboard or the freezer, I'll eat them. So I try to avoid bringing sugary foods into my house, and then I don't even think about them (er, mostly).

Here's how my brain works: I go to the cabinet to look for a snack when I'm feeling slightly hungry. There's a full fruit basket, but I dig through the cabinet, which is packed full with grains, dried beans, canned beans, and trail mix. And I think, "There's nothing to eat." So I'll go get a piece of fruit. And after I eat the piece of fruit, I'll feel glad that I did. But if there was something in the cabinet that was much fattier, sweeter, or more convenient, I would've eaten it in a minute. When you eliminate the options you're trying to avoid, you set yourself up to make better choices. It might not be what you want in the moment, but you'll be glad you did it in the end.

Put Your Foot in the Door. There's a strategy for sales and persuasion called "foot in the door" in which once someone agrees to a small purchase or request, they'll be more likely to agree with follow-up requests of a similar nature. Studies have been done for decades on this strategy, and it consistently appears to work.[15]

A similarly important phenomenon to change-making is labeling and self-identity. Researchers have found that individuals who have been assigned a specific label perceived themselves to be like, and behave consistent with, that label.[16] In one study, researchers called homes, asking to speak with the woman of the house. They shared with the women information about the work of the Red Cross. They closed some of the calls by saying they wished more people were as interested in their "fellow man" as the woman with whom they were talking. Later, following up to thank them for being a *supporter* made the women significantly more likely to say they would volunteer for the Red Cross than individuals who had not received such a call and been labeled as a *supporter*.[17] I've personally experienced this phenomenon when, for example a colleague tells me I'm hard-working or effective at my job. It makes me want to work harder and consider ways to be more effective.

In one study, researchers found that by reminding participants about their previous environmentally friendly behavior, their attitude toward environmentally friendly actions improved, making them more open to requests to adopt additional behaviors to help the environment. "The cueing of common ecological behaviors leads participants to choose environmentally friendly products with greater frequency, and even to use scrap paper more efficiently," the researchers concluded. They even found that the subjects wrote smaller to use less of the paper provided![18]

So what can we learn from these studies? And how can we apply that to our efforts to make dietary changes? First get your foot in the door. You don't have to become vegan overnight (or ever). Try Meatless Monday—or being vegan before 6 p.m., as former *New York Times'* columnist Mark Bittman suggests. You'll likely find that once you get started making some of these changes they become a part of your normal routine.

Make Change Part of Your Identity. Dr. Esherick knows how important the role of identity plays in behavior change. She shared the following personal example: "After my beloved dog of twelve years, Mogli, died suddenly, I sought out volunteer opportunities to help animals as a way to get through my grief. To learn about the different ways I might help animals, I attended an animal welfare conference. When I learned that the majority of suffering and mistreated animals were farmed animals (accounting for about 99 percent of all the animals suffering in the world), and that I could help hundreds of animals a year just by not eating them, I stopped eating animals. My identity as an animal lover helped me change my eating habits. As someone who loved animals, I could no longer justify eating them and contributing to their suffering on factory farms.

"Now, when I am tempted to eat meat or other animal products, I ask myself the 'Who am I?' question, and what would someone like me do in this situation? I remind myself of my core values, of what's important to me: I'm someone who cares about animals, and because of this I do not want to contribute to the unnecessary suffering and abuse of animals. Because factory farming causes extreme and unnecessary suffering, I am not someone who wants to support this industry and its way of treating animals."[19]

As with the prospective Red Cross donors who were told they were the type of person who donated, when we give ourselves labels, we will be more likely to consider ourselves the kind of person who acts according to that label—and we will make decisions accordingly.

So give yourself a label and make that change a part of who you are. Whatever your reason is for choosing meat*less*, own it—slap that label on! Are you an animal lover and you don't want to contribute to the suffering of animals on factory farms? There you go: you're an animal lover. When you make decisions, consider this: *What would an animal lover do in this situation?* Are you a healthy person who wants to stay fit? When choosing what to eat at a restaurant, ask yourself, *Which of these options would a healthy person choose?* Are you an environmentalist who wants to lighten your footprint on the planet? Make your decision based on what an environmentalist would do. Or consider yourself a meat reducer, a flexitarian, a vegetarian, or a vegan. These labels will help shape your self-perception and guide your decisions.

MeatLess Movements

By now you've probably discerned that there's no right or wrong approach. Maybe like Dr. Esherick you're inspired to try to become vegan and want to jump in headfirst. Or perhaps you'd like to dip your toes in the water and make small changes. Whatever you feel is the best path for you, there's a roadmap for getting there. The following are just a couple of options:

Meatless Monday

In 2003, the Johns Hopkins Bloomberg School of Public Health teamed up with the Monday Campaigns, a public health effort started by retired advertising guru Sid Lerner, to begin Meatless Monday. Lerner, who had been a successful ad man decades before *Mad Men*'s Don Draper gave us a behind the scenes look at the advertising world, directed the creative team behind the famous "Don't squeeze the Charmin" commercials, popularized over the course of two decades.

A long-time health advocate, Lerner and his wife, Helaine, wanted to devote their retirement to improving public health. Having heard that the US Surgeon General had recommended lowering meat consumption by 15 percent to reduce the intake of saturated fat, Lerner realized that 15 percent equals roughly one day a week.

Knowing what a proper portion size is can be difficult for many of us. So as Lerner told Fox News, "You can't take 15 percent of every spoon or every plate or every meal, but you can take it out of the 21 meals you eat a week, which is one day's meals."[20] Lerner's team did some research and determined that Monday is the day of the week when people are ripe to make healthy changes. We often eat or drink too much on the weekend and can think, "I'm going to start fresh on Monday." It's like being able to do a New Year's resolution without having to wait until the start of the year.

> **Did you know?**
>
> Meatless Monday was initiated by the US Food Administration during World War I as a resource conservation campaign. Back then 13 million families pledged to reduce consumption of key staples to assist the war effort.

To put the icing on the cake, Lerner remembered a World War I campaign by the US Food Administration that encouraged Americans to go meat-free one day a week (to do their part to conserve resources during the war when food was scarce). The conservation campaign was brought back during World War II for the same reasons. A half a century later the effort was reborn as Meatless Monday, with Lerner's prime motivation to help fight other wars: the ones against chronic, preventable disease and climate change. Since its re-launch, millions of individuals have vowed to take a holiday from meat on Mondays to get their week off to a healthy start.

The program started with promotion from bloggers and grassroots advocates. Within a few years, media icons such as Michael Pollan, author of several *New York Time*s bestselling food books, and later celebrity supporters such as Paul McCartney (who has his own "Meat-Free Mondays" campaign), Oprah Winfrey, and Gwyneth Paltrow professed their Meatless Monday pledges publicly.

Today, there are thousands of schools, hospitals, colleges, and universities supporting the program, because of the efforts of organizations like The Monday Campaigns and the Humane Society of the United States. Restaurants, including steakhouses, offer Meatless Monday specials. And entire cities—Washington, DC, San Francisco, Los Angeles, and Cleveland—have promoted Meatless Monday by passing resolutions and proclamations endorsing the concept. Meatless Monday is now a global program, active in thirty-five countries, from South Korea and Kuwait to South Africa and the Philippines.[21] For more information on Meatless Monday, visit www.meatlessmonday.com

Flexing Your Diet

Maybe you're ready to go beyond Meatless Monday. Another great program that encourages a mostly plant-based diet is the "Flexitarian" diet, in which people eat vegetarian most of the time, with some flexibility. It's become so popular that Compass Group, which operates dining halls in tens of thousands of corporate cafeterias, colleges, universities, and even the US Senate, promotes flexitarian eating at locations across the United States.

Mark Bittman, former food columnist for the *New York Times*, made the concept of being a part-time vegan easy and popular with his book *Vegan Before Six* published in 2013. The respected food policy analyst and author of numerous cookbooks wrote of how he was overweight, on the verge of diabetes, suffering from knee pain and high cholesterol. His doctor gave him two options: eat a plant-based diet or go on medication that he'd likely have to be on for life.

As someone whose very livelihood revolved around food, the thought of either of those options was unappealing, to say the least. So Bittman, who said he'd always enjoyed beans and tofu but also loved bacon and burgers, decided to compromise and become a flexitarian. However, he needed some boundaries. He decided that he'd eat plant-based foods two-thirds of the time (for breakfast and lunch). After that, he'd eat his typical meals that weren't as healthy. If he wanted to eat meat, eggs, or dairy for dinner, he could, though in moderation. He dubbed his diet *Vegan Before Six.*[22]

Within a month, he had lost 15 pounds. After two months of this plan, his blood sugar and cholesterol were down. His cholesterol dropped from 240 to 180! After four months of eating vegan before six, Bittman was down 35 pounds. He said he weighed less than he had in thirty years. Following this plan also led to some changes in how he ate dinner too, making these lifestyle changes lasting.

Flip Your Plate

Menus of Change is an annual conference assembled by the Culinary Institute of America and the Harvard School of Public Health, and is attended by chefs, public health experts, and representatives from some of the world's biggest food companies.[23] The conference emphasizes the importance of reducing animal products and getting more plant-based foods on Americans' plates. Backed by Dr. Walter Willet, chairman of Harvard's School of Public Health, the conference's Principles of Healthy, Sustainable Menus recommend moving nuts and legumes to the center of the plate and leveraging globally-inspired plant-based recipes and meal offerings.[24]

Chefs and foodservice providers are responding to this rally cry with a host of novel approaches. University of California, Berkeley students enjoy plant-forward meals at Brown's—A California Café. At this campus favorite, guests can opt for the less-meat "Flipped Plate," with seasonal plant choices of brown rice, caramelized onion and parsley pilaf; roasted broccoli with cumin; and house-made hummus with paprika pita chips and an entrée. This includes plant-based options such as root vegetable gratin and grilled portabella mushroom caps. Or guest can go totally vegan with a sampler plate featuring all-vegetable options as the stars of the dish.

Others chefs and individuals are going back to their roots by making meat a garnish rather than the center of the plate, using it to flavor foods, or doing meat-vegetable blends, like a meat-mushroom blended burger. These examples represent just a couple of options for flipping the conventional plate and getting on a path to meat*less*.

Be the Tortoise

Although meat consumption is declining, the number of Americans who report being vegetarian or vegan remains relatively steady. Research from Faunalytics, in 2014, found that most vegetarians who stuck with the diet had made the transition gradually.[25] Though we would all love to make immediate changes in our diets, especially once we've learned about the important reasons for doing so, there's a compelling case to be made for taking baby steps.

You're probably familiar with the classic Aesop fable about the tortoise and the hare. The hare taunts the tortoise who challenges him to race in what would seem to be a rather unfair competition. The hare starts out strong, leaving his competitor far behind. Certain of his victory, the hare decides to take a snooze along the way. When he wakes up, he learns the slow as molasses tortoise has already won the race. Thus the saying goes, "Slow and steady wins the race." Some people might be able to move to a plant-based diet overnight; others may choose never to do so. If you want to win the race though, consider going slow and steady like the tortoise. Whatever method works for you, you gotta tie up your sneakers and get started.

Dining Out

Eating meat*less* out can be easy, but it's even easier when you plan ahead and do some research. Once you get the hang of it, it becomes second nature.

We learned from the psychological studies that we tend to stick with the default, so a key is to make the default the healthy, meat-free option. If your default lunch option with teammates has been a fast food hamburger, change that. How about making your new lunch destination Chipotle, where you can get a burrito with spicy tofu Sofritas, or Burger King, which has a veggie burger? Most restaurants offer meat-free foods! Think about vegetable pizzas, sandwiches, salads, pastas, and more! Though it's easy to find these types of food, here's a list of specific options at chain restaurants to get you started. New options are appearing on menus all of the time—these options are just some examples at the time of writing this book. Note that not all of these are totally vegan by default, though many can customize the dishes to be so.

- Burger King offers a veggie burger at all US locations.

- The Cheesecake Factory offers many options, including pasta dishes, wraps, and a veggie burger made with brown rice, farro, couscous, mushrooms, black beans, and onions.

- Chili's offers a black bean burger patty and assorted salads that can be customized to be meatless.

- Chipotle: build a burrito, tacos, or bowls with its tofu-based Sofritas, or opt for beans, rice, grilled vegetables, and guacamole.

- Denny's offers bagels, oatmeal, English muffins, grits, and a veggie burger.

- Friendly's Ice Cream offers a vegan Gardein burger.

- Fuddrucker's offers a veggie burger.

- Johnny Rockets offers a veggie burger, the "Streamliner."

- Little Caesar's: its regular crust and sauce are vegan, so add your favorite vegetable toppings for an easy cheese-free pizza.

- Moe's: burritos, bowls, and tacos with your favorite ingredients, including a spicy tofu.

- Noodles & Co. offers tofu as the protein for any menu item, including the Indonesian Peanut Sauté and the Japanese Pan Noodles.

- Olive Garden offers a number of meatless pasta dishes.

- P.F. Chang's offers a number of vegan options such as lettuce wraps, kung pao bean curd (tofu), Chang's bean curd, coconut-curry vegetables, ma po bean curd, Singapore street noodles, and more. You can also make most meat items on the menu vegetarian by substituting tofu.

- Panera Bread offers a black bean soup and a soba noodle bowl with edamame.

- Papa John's: its sauce and original hand-tossed dough are vegan, so add your favorite vegetable toppings for a delicious cheese-free pizza. Plus, its garlic sauce is vegan too!

- Qdoba: build a burrito, taco, or salad bowl, or enjoy the tortilla soup.

- Red Robin: a veggie burger can be used for any burger option on the menu, and it offers a hummus plate.

- Ruby Tuesday offers a veggie trio combo, allowing you to choose three sides to create a meal and a Garden Bar where you can build your own salad.

(*Continues*)

(*Continued*)

- Souplantation and Sweet Tomatoes: build your own salad and add on prepared salads. They often have several vegan selections, like dill and Dijon potato salad, lemon linguine with fresh basil, kale and harvest salad with toasted almonds, whole wheat spicy Asian peanut noodles, Santa Fe black bean chili, roasted ratatouille, and baked potatoes which you can pile high with your favorite toppings.

- Starbucks offers a Hearty Veggie and Brown Rice Salad Bowl, oatmeal, as well as almond, coconut, and soy milk for beverages.

- Subway offers a veggie sub and, at some US locations, offers a falafel sandwich, black bean sandwich, or Malibu garden sandwich.

- Taco Bell: from bean and seven layer burritos to taco salad, you can easily eat meat*less* by asking to substitute beans for meat on menu options and requesting no dairy.

- White Castle: veggie sliders are available at all its four hundred locations nationwide.

Travel 'Round the World— Restaurant by Restaurant

International restaurants—from Italian to Ethiopian—offer an abundance of delicious, healthy, meat-free fare!

- Chinese: Almost every town has a Chinese restaurant where you can find loads of options. From vegetable chow mein to sweet and sour tofu to Szechuan string beans, there are typically options listed on the menu, or you can ask to substitute meat with tofu.

- Ethiopian: Most Ethiopian restaurants offer meatless dishes such as stews made from lentils, peas, chickpeas, cabbage, greens, and more, slow cooked in savory-spiced sauces.

- Indian: With India's large population of vegetarians, it's no wonder meatless fare is found in abundance at Indian restaurants. Try chana masala (spiced chickpeas simmered in tomatoes), aloo gobi (potatoes, cauliflower, and spices), eggplant bharta (roasted, spiced eggplant), aloo saag (spinach and potatoes cooked with spices), or crispy Bombay potatoes. And don't forget the roti, a delicious wheat flatbread!

- Italian: One word: pasta. Most Italian restaurants offer a host of meatless options, but if you don't see anything on the menu, ask the chef to cook up some noodles and vegetables tossed with garlic and olive oil or a vegetable pizza.

- Mediterranean: Classic Mediterranean dishes of hummus, falafel (crispy chickpea patties often served stuffed in pita bread), baba ganoush (roasted eggplant dip), and dolmas (grape leaves stuffed with rice and vegetables) are traditionally meatless. Order a mezze platter with a side of warm pita bread for a filling meal.

- Mexican: Most Mexican restaurants have an array of meatless options, yet some use lard or stock from animal sources in their beans. After checking how they cook their beans, substitute beans for meat in any meal, such as enchiladas verde, tacos, burritos, or a fiesta taco salad.

- Japanese: Sushi is one of my personal favorites. Although most people associate sushi with raw fish, the term actually refers to the rice.[26] Any sushi restaurant can make colorful vegetable rolls, making it an easy option when traveling. Order your favorite fillings like avocado, cucumber, carrots, sweet potato, and asparagus. And if you're feeling like trying something more exotic, go for pickled burdock root or kanpyo (squash).

- Thai: Most towns now have Thai restaurants that serve delicious noodle dishes like pad Thai, curries made with coconut milk and vegetables, and pad see-ew (pan fried rice noodles with broccoli, cabbage, carrots).

5

So What the Heck Do I Eat?

K en Botts, a thirty-year food service industry veteran, has spent most of his life feeding people. He attributes his career path to his mother. "You will always have a job if you work in food service because people always have to eat," she told him. So he got a job washing dishes in a restaurant when he was fifteen years old. Since then, he's managed and trained dozens of people; opened, closed, and owned restaurants; and worked in college and university food service.[1]

At the University of North Texas (UNT), in the small town of Denton, Botts wore many hats—from marketing and working with the chefs to developing recipes and designing new concepts. In 2011, Botts was tasked with a project that put UNT on the map in a big way and changed the direction of his life: creating the nation's first vegan dining hall.

UNT's decision stemmed from student requests. From inviting students to share comments during student advisory meetings and using conventional feedback methods to looking at national trends in colleges and university food service, the writing was on the wall: students want healthy options, and many who don't consider themselves vegetarian or vegan still want to eat meat-free foods.

UNT wanted to satisfy students by giving them what they wanted. In response, it opened a vegan dining hall, Mean Greens, in the fall of 2011. The dining hall's popularity exceeded expectations. The school saw a double-digit increase in cafeteria participation—the industry's term for number of patrons buying meals—and unprecedented press coverage.

"Nine out of ten of the students who come to Mean Greens aren't vegetarian or vegan; they come because the food tastes good," Botts shared.

One of his favorite news stories came from *ABC News*, entitled, "Adios, A-Meat-Gos . . . Texas College Caf Goes Vegan."[2] Reporters said what everyone was thinking, *a vegan cafeteria . . . in Texas?*

Botts is now a food policy manager with the Humane Society of the United States, where he helps colleges and universities nationwide replicate the type of success he was able to execute at UNT.

Meat-free eating has really hit its stride, with its popularity swelling from beef country to both coasts. The restaurant industry is responding too. *USA Today* wrote about this trend, saying vegetables are shifting to the center of the plate.[3] No longer are they relegated to the side, soaked in butter, and overcooked, largely an afterthought. Instead they're playing center stage. French chef Alain Ducasse, who has more Michelin stars than any other chef on the planet, reopened his world-renowned restaurant at the Hôtel Plaza Athénée in Paris with a vegetable-centric menu. He told news agency Agence France-Presse, "The planet has increasingly rare resources so we have to consume more ethically, more fairly."[6]

> **Did you know?**
>
> Eating meatless can help you save money. A pound of lentils at Walmart costs $1.54.[4] A pound of beef costs $3.97.[5]

Haute or Not?

Chef Alexandra (Alex) Bury grew up in Alaska, where food options were limited. Venison was easy to come by, but fresh vegetables? Not so much. As a child, she'd receive oranges for Christmas—that's how rare fresh fruit was.

Bury eventually left Alaska and attended the Culinary Institute of America (CIA) in upstate New York, where she learned gourmet cooking.

"You name it, I ate it," she said. "Foie gras. Veal. It was all game. My specialty was baby lamb brains."

After graduating from the CIA, Bury cooked in kitchens worldwide—San Francisco, Paris, New Orleans, and, yes, even Alaska.[7] She became vegan after watching a slaughterhouse video, though continued cooking meat for another year, and eventually opened an all-vegan restaurant in California's wine country that received critical acclaim.

Bury went to work as a chef instructor for several years at Dr. John McDougall's Health and Medical Center which offers a ten-day live-in program to help patients suffering from hypertension, type-2 diabetes, indigestion, constipation, and other ailments learn about plant-based eating. She talks about the seemingly magical transformation that patients were able to make after just a few days of being there and changing their diets to eat plant-based foods.

"Inevitably," she says, "someone would lose their wedding ring over the course of the 10-day program because the weight was coming off them so quickly." It was a joy for her to see people who had arrived in wheelchairs, unable to walk more than a few steps, get up and start moving on their own after eating healthier foods.

Bury's specialty is helping people new to meatless eating make simple transitions to ensure their success. She's done cooking demonstrations for corporations interested in helping their employees make better choices and at community centers for people interested in making dietary changes. Most of the time her audience consists of people who are brand new to meatless eating.

Bury starts her cooking demos with an exclusive top-secret recipe that I'll share with you, with her permission. Go ahead and give it a try: Take two heaping tablespoons of butter and place in a bowl. Then take two heaping teaspoons of salt and coat the butter with the salt. That's it! Look appetizing? Probably not.

The Hard Stuff:
Top Ten Frequently Asked Questions

No, really: What *do* I eat? Variety is the spice of life, and most people find that when they start eating more plant-based foods, they actually find all kinds of new flavors and meals and products they love but might not have otherwise tried. The world of produce is as colorful as a rainbow, with incredible—and healthy!—fruits and veggies galore. Plus there are really innovative and delicious new products coming out all the time—cheeses made from almonds, yogurt made from coconuts, and meat-free chicken made from pea and carrot protein that has the same taste and texture of chicken, and so much more. Plus, give ethnic foods a shot—Ethiopian, Vietnamese, Thai, Mexican, Chinese, and most other international fare feature meat-free options. Adding in these types of products and meals will open you up to a whole wide world of foods that you may not have ever even known about before.

1. WHAT ABOUT PROTEIN?

Whether you're reducing or eliminating meat from your diet, nutritionists and scientists agree that even vegetarians and vegans get plenty of protein (and, in fact, people with meat at the center of their plate at every meal likely eat an unhealthy amount of it). Many of the foods you're already familiar with pack a protein punch—beans, grains, peanut butter, lentils, and more. Or try tofu and tempeh, which (like raw chicken) essentially just take on the flavors of whatever spices and sauces they're cooked with. Then there are all the meat-free meats, such as those mentioned above— veggie burgers and chickenless nuggets, meat-free wings, bacon, ground beef crumbles, deli slices, and more. All of these products have at least as much protein—and in many cases, more protein—as their animal-based counterparts. For more on getting protein and other key nutrients, see Chapter 6.

2. HOW AM I SUPPOSED TO COOK WITHOUT MEAT, MILK, AND EGGS?

This is the burning question most everyone has when thinking about eating meatless. When Botts helped open Mean Greens, he worked closely with Chef Wanda White, a classically trained French pastry chef.

"The first question she asked me was, 'Ken, how am I supposed to cook without meat, milk, and eggs?'"

The answer, Botts explained, was easy. "You probably eat a lot of meatless meals already and don't think much about it," he told her. "Bean and rice burritos, bean chilis, eggplant parmesan, mushroom ravioli, avocado sushi rolls, even peanut butter and jelly! They're foods most people eat all the time, and they're already meatless."[8]

3. HOW CAN I EAT MEATLESS ON A SMALL BUDGET?

Actually, meat-free eating tends to be the more affordable way to eat. Beans and legumes, lentils and tofu, whole grains and vegetables: because these foods are less resource-intensive to produce than meat (which requires massive amounts of land, feed crops, water, processing, and more), they're also less expensive to buy. If you're on a budget, probably skip the plant-based meats and focus on these good-for-you foods.

4. CAN I EAT MEATLESS AND BE AN ATHLETE?

Absolutely! In fact, meat-free eating is taking the field of athletics by storm! You can barely open a fitness magazine or read the sports pages these days without seeing an article about a vegan football player, professional fighter, or body builder. Check out The300PoundVegan.com—the website of former NFL linebacker (and vegan) David Carter; it's packed full of useful information on meat-free eating for athletes.

Former professional Ironman Brendan Brazier's *Thrive* books series and website also offer valuable tips and suggestions for supporting and enhancing athletic performance on a plant-based diet. Visit Brendanbrazier.com.

5. CAN I BE MEATLESS WHILE PREGNANT, AND CAN CHILDREN EAT MEAT-FREE?

Avoiding animal products while pregnant has always been good for both mother and child—as has feeding your kids a healthy, well-balanced diet that's lower in meat and dairy products. In fact, the late Dr. Benjamin Spock, arguably the most influential pediatrician of all time, advised that children and parents stick to a vegetarian diet free from all dairy products

(Continues)

after the age of two. "We now know that there are harmful effects of a meaty diet," says Dr. Spock in the last edition of his world-famous book, *Baby and Child Care*. "Children can get plenty of protein and iron from vegetables, beans, and other plant foods that avoid the fat and cholesterol that are in animal products." As for dairy foods, Dr. Spock says, "Other calcium sources offer many advantages that dairy products do not have."[9]

6. WHAT DO I DO WHEN INVITED TO SOMEONE'S HOUSE FOR DINNER, OR FOR HOLIDAYS?

Nowadays, meat-free (and dairy-free) eating has become so common that you should be able to find an array of options at any dinner party. Though just to be safe—and courteous!—what many people choose to do is call or e-mail the host a few days beforehand just to drop a polite note letting him or her know about your dietary choices. And for holidays, if you think about a typical, say, Thanksgiving or Christmas spread, you'll realize that many of your favorite holiday foods are already meat-free: cranberry sauce and stuffing (if it wasn't in the bird!), beautiful salads and roasted vegetables, breads galore, vegetable dishes like green beans and sweet potatoes, and so many more.

7. IF WE DIDN'T EAT THEM, WHAT WOULD HAPPEN TO THE ANIMALS?

Farm animals exist only because we breed them into existence for the purpose of eating them (or their milk or eggs). The less demand for their products there is, the fewer of these animals will be bred. And that's a good thing, as most farm animals live lives of complete deprivation on factory farms—where they're often crammed into tiny cages and crates, or (in the case of chickens) bred to grow so fat so fast that their legs may literally break underneath them.

8. WHAT IF I JUST LOVE STEAK TOO MUCH TO GO MEAT-FREE?

Then eat steak but purchase it from producers who adhere to higher animal welfare standards, such as those who are part of the Global Animal Partnership program. Many people choose to be entirely vegan or vegetarian, though countless others are simply reducing the amount of meat they eat and replacing it with products from those who treat their animals more humanely—and there's a place for everyone at the table when it comes to plant-forward diets. There are no hard and fast rules to this stuff, so just do what feels right and you're guaranteed to feel better.

9. HOW CAN I SURVIVE WITHOUT BACON?

There are so many great animal-free bacon products out there today! From meatless bacons that have the salt and fat we crave, and sizzle up like the animal-based counterpart to bacon bit toppings, there are vegan bacons available! But, like the steak answer above, if you think you just have to have bacon once in a while, then so be it. You can eat meat-free all or much of the time, without being so purist about it that you pine after your favorite foods.

10. HOW DO I DEAL WITH FRIENDS, FAMILY, AND OTHERS WHO AREN'T SUPPORTIVE OR DON'T UNDERSTAND?

Be a positive, friendly voice on these issues. Food is wrapped up in all kinds of personal issues—memory and culture, family, and identity. So some people may just not "get it." The best advice is not to be pushy about your own diet (or theirs) and let the people around you find their own journey toward healthier eating. Be a positive example and others will no doubt follow your lead.

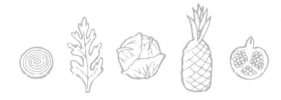

The point to this exercise is that all that fat, all that salt—that's what we're eating when we eat cheese pizza, fast food hamburgers, and fried chicken sandwiches. We just don't realize it because it's disguised in the cheese and meat. It's not our fault. We're genetically wired to crave fat, salt, and sugar.

As David Linden—Ph.D. and author of *The Compass of Pleasure: How Our Brains Make Fatty Foods, Orgasm, Exercise, Marijuana, Generosity, Vodka, Learning, and Gambling Feel So Good*—explains, "In many locations intermittent famines were regular occurrences, so when energy-dense foods containing fat and sugar were available, it made sense to gorge on them to establish a body fat reserve for anticipated hard times."[10] Of course we don't need to do that these days, and in fact we're getting way too many of those foods. However, we're "hardwired from birth to like certain tastes and smells, most notably those of sugar and fat, but also salt."[11]

Don't underestimate how much we eat and how much we love fat, salt, and sugar! And be kind to yourself. You're unlikely to be satisfied if you go from eating chicken nuggets and French fries for lunch to brown rice, beans, and broccoli. But if you make gradual changes, as you get healthier, your taste buds will change; it will become easier to make those adjustments. For starters though, incorporating more meatless meals into your life is a good step in the right direction.

So back to what to eat. Where should we begin? Set yourself up for success by setting a realistic goal. When you meet that goal, celebrate it. Choose the best goal for you. Start with one meal at a time. There's no one-size-fits-all plan; there are many ways for you to get started (see "Daily MeatLess Goals"), certainly far more than I'm offering here—just pick the one that works for you.

Third Time's a Charm

"I'm done eating meat," was Anthony Williams' reaction after watching the film *Super Size Me*, in 2005. A then-recent law school graduate studying for the bar exam, Williams was an educated man. Yet this documentary featuring Morgan Spurlock on a thirty-day regimen of breakfast, lunch, and dinner from McDonald's educated him in a whole different way. His world was rocked by what he saw: Spurlock getting sicker and sicker as the month went on as a result of his diet high in meat and animal protein. He told his then-girlfriend (now wife), Keiko, he was going vegetarian and did it cold turkey.

"Every time I thought about eating meat, I thought about the animals," he recalls.

He stuck with his meatless diet until the end of that year when he visited his fiancée's family in Japan. Anthony and Keiko were both worried about the cultural acceptance of showing up at someone's home and refusing to eat what was served or imposing on them, so he slowly added meat to his diet. By the spring of 2006 when they got married, he was back to eating meat—a full carnivore as he described himself.

Eight years later, in the fall of 2014, Williams was making a transition in his work. He and Keiko had three kids and he was relocating the family from Sacramento to Southern California. One evening while he was in Southern California and Keiko was up north in Sacramento with the kids, she called him and said, "Honey, we're not eating meat anymore." She'd watched the documentary *Food, Inc.* and realized what a huge impact animal agribusiness has not just on animals, but also on the environment, and our health. One of their favorite things to do as a family was to cook on the grill on Sundays and dine on the pork chops, hamburgers, and lamb chops, which had perfectly seasoned his prized grill, throughout the week. They decided to give the grill away and significantly cut back on meat consumption. They did cut back for a while, but as soon as it got difficult, such as making meal choices for the kids on busy school nights, they went back to their old habits.

In the spring of 2016, Williams attended a gala for the Humane Society of the United States, benefitting the organization's work protecting farm animals. The evening's entertainment—featuring performances by singer Ke$ha, Steven Tyler of Aerosmith, and Leona Lewis—was peppered with information on the abuses animals endure on factory farms. Celebrities like Moby and Kate Mara encouraged attendees to consider going meat-free or even trying Meatless Monday.

Daily Meal Meat*less* Goals

- **Switch your breakfasts to plant-based.** This one is a cinch, right? Skip the bacon, sausage, and eggs and opt instead for fluffy blueberry pancakes. Try Belgian waffles, oatmeal with fresh berries, a fruit smoothie, breakfast burritos, cereal with soy milk topped with fruit, or if you just want something simple, toast with jam, peanut or almond butter, or toast with avocado and a sprinkle of salt.

- **Switch your lunches to plant-based.** Whether you brown bag it or you eat lunch on the run, don't let your afternoon meals slow you down. If you pack your lunch, try a rainbow hummus wrap stuffed with roasted red peppers and fresh salad mix, a hearty salad topped with beans and a hunk of bread on the side, a hero made with Tofurky deli slices, or a simple peanut butter and jelly sandwich. There are loads of plant-based burritos and soups to make your brown-bagged lunch something to look forward to. Amy's offers delicious frozen burritos and meals as well as canned soups and chilis. Sweet Earth Natural Foods frozen wraps, like the Curry Tiger and the Kyoto, are inspired by international flavors. Even Hormel—maker of SPAM—has a canned vegetarian chili!

- **Explore on-the-go options.** Of course, many of us have to eat on the road. Try some of the meatless options listed in Chapter 4, such as a veggie burger at Burger King, Denny's, Johnny Rockets, White Castle, Red Robin, or Friendly's. Or swing by Chipotle for a vegetable or "Sofritas" burrito—a spicy blend of braised tofu and peppers. Note that not all the aforementioned are vegan. However, I've found that when asked, almost every restaurant can make something vegan and oftentimes the vegan guest will end up with the most delectable meal at the table if the chef is invited to make something special.

- **Switch your comfort items to plant-based.** If you have a daily latte or cappuccino, try it with soy milk, coconut milk, or almond milk instead of cows' milk. If your day wouldn't be complete without a bowl of ice cream, try one of the many incredible dairy-free varieties made out of cashew cream, almond milk, rice milk, soy milk, or coconut milk. If you're handy in the kitchen, experiment with vegan baking.

- **Make a favorite meal meatless.** Choose one favorite meal a week to make meatless, one you currently make on a regular basis. That can be your standby recipe.

- **Go meatless every Monday.** Then go meatless every Monday and Wednesday. And gradually increase it from there if you feel comfortable.

- **Eat vegan before 6 p.m. like Mark Bittman.** Keep the momentum going throughout the evening if you feel up to it.

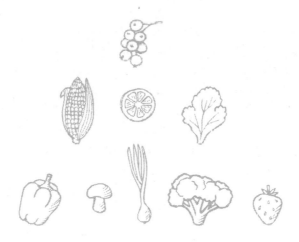

Williams left inspired to try to do something about it.

The next day he spoke with his family. He told them about Meatless Monday, which he learned about at the gala. His six-year-old son told him he knew about Meatless Monday—that his school participates. "How about this?" Williams posed. "Let's not try a cold turkey thing like we did before. Let's do one meal each day with no meat and one day a week with no meat. It won't change the world, but it's relatively easy." They all agreed.

For the Williams family, a Meatless Monday plus a meat-free meal once a day was a doable goal. And it's working for them. For Anthony, it's easy, and he finds that he's gone beyond the one day a week holiday from meat.

"There's probably one meal every three days where I'm eating meat," he says. "So I've totally exceeded the goal."

This new approach allows the family the structure to stay on course with a meatless day a week, but without the rigidity of feeling like they've failed and have to reset if they eat meat.

"We're having fun cooking together and trying new things. I'm no longer just the Sunday grill guy; I'm a little more involved in meal prep," Williams said.

They experiment with new recipes. Keiko makes a meatloaf with tofu that Williams loves. It's now one of his favorite meals. The whole family was blown away by an avocado taco recipe. Dinner, the meal at which they used to eat the most meat, is vegetarian roughly four nights a week.

Williams reports that even when Keiko includes meat in a meal, she uses significantly less than she did before. "For example, if she prepares spaghetti with meat sauce, she'll use, say, half a pound of ground beef rather than a pound. As a result, she said we buy probably 50 to 75 percent less meat than we did before."

A runner who averages about 15 miles a week, Williams has found that he has more energy and physical stamina with his new approach to eating.

"When I run, even if I haven't run in a while, I'm finding I'm not as fatigued or winded as I used to be."

This flexible approach works for Williams because it solves the all-or-nothing problem for him.

"I'm not that kind of person," he said. "Once I fell off the wagon, I stayed off the wagon."

Now, though, when he approaches a meal choice, he looks for a vegetarian option that works for him and chooses that. Williams's advice to anyone who wants to eat more meatless meals is to "do what works for you." There's an adage that the way to eat an elephant—solve a big problem—is one small bite at a time. The bite-size approach has proven to work for Williams and many others, and may well work for you too.[12]

Tofu or Not Tofu: That Is the Question

Speaking of elephants, let's go ahead and get this one out of the room: when people think of vegetarian meals, they often think of tofu. Just because you're eating more meat-free meals doesn't mean you have to eat tofu (poor old, maligned tofu), though many people enjoy it as a nutritional powerhouse. But what exactly is tofu? It's a protein-packed food that's been eaten in Asia for millennia. Ben Franklin introduced it to America. He sent some soybeans and a recipe for tofu back from London in the 1700s, calling it "a kind of cheese made in China from a little bean."[13]

Today, there are many varieties of tofu, and it's important to know the differences. Silken tofu is unpressed (that is, still full of water) and thus very delicate. It's often used in desserts or for baking. Firm tofu, on the other hand, has had much of the water pressed from it and thus takes on a much denser, firmer texture. This tofu you'd use to make savory entrees. Although tofu on its own is bland and flavorless—just like a piece of raw chicken or hunk of ground beef

Did you know?

Meatless meats have been consumed for centuries, tracing their roots all the way back to 1300 AD in China.[14] Today the US plant-based meat market is valued at $854 million and is expected to reach $1.1 billion by 2020.[15]

would be—its beauty is that, like those meats, it soaks up the flavors of marinades and sauces. (Remember my story about eating plain raw tofu? Bad idea, bad idea.)

Chef Bury likens it to a raw chicken breast: "You wouldn't just eat a plain chicken breast, unless you were on a bland diet prescribed by your doctor," she says.

It's an a-ha moment for many who've tried tofu to less than satisfactory results. Tofu should be considered a vehicle for flavor. When we marinate it, soak it in sauces, or pureé it with seasonings for a ricotta, it can become a delicious, healthy, and important staple of our diets. But eating less meat doesn't mean you're required to get a tofu frequent eater card; there are plenty of other sources of protein and hearty staples.

The Meat of Plant-based Meats

Plant-based meats and cheeses are popping up everywhere. According to *Global Meat News* (yes, there's a publication for everything!), the plant-based meat sector will grow by more than 8 percent annually by 2020.[16] Not every vegan or meat reducer loves them, and I like some and not others. My point here is, these meats may or may not be for you and perhaps some are and others aren't. You probably have a favorite chicken nugget brand or hamburger joint and some you don't like as much. The same will be true of plant-based meats. Keep in mind that these meatless meats and cheeses won't be exact replicas of the hamburgers and cheeses you love. And they're not all amazing. But many are so good and so meaty you may be fooled. Plus, they're a convenient and often easy way to round out a meal, fulfill a craving for comfort foods, or fit in at a cookout.

The Big Cheese

Speaking of cheese, there are a number of plant-based cheese companies popping up. From Field Roast's Chao slices to Daiya, which has a line of shredded toppings like mozzarella and Monterey Jack to melt on pizzas as well as slices and cream cheese spreads, to Kite Hill, a gourmet variety found at Whole Foods Market, to Mikoyo's Kitchen's artisan cultured nut cheeses founded by cookbook author and chef Miyoko Schinner. More and more, purveyors are pioneering this new sector and to great success.

Of Miyoko's cheeses, Jonathan Kauffman, food writer for the *San Francisco Chronicle* wrote, "Schinner's cheeses do have tanginess and significant complexity. They deliver huge hits of umami, that mouth-filling savoriness that lures you into scattering an extra quarter-cup of Parmesan across your bowl of pasta."[17] Schinner has even created a pizza-worthy mozzarella and a European-style cultured butter.

I don't want to oversimplify this. If you're thinking, "I could never live without cheese," I have two things to share. First, you don't have to. Second, you can.

Also, I can relate. I remember attending my first ever vegan holiday party, in 1997, and uttering those very words. You know what? I live without cheese; I don't miss it or want it and even if I did, the amazing benefits of living without it dramatically outweigh the momentary pleasure I might have gotten from eating it.

When I'm craving something cheesy I make a batch of cashew cheese which can be made in minutes in a high powered blender and pour it over nachos or eat it in macaroni and cheese [see recipe page 189]. I'll buy a bag of dairy-free mozzarella and pile it on a pizza. Or I'll get some crackers and dive into a round of vegan soft cheese. Craving = satisfied.

If you're in the camp of a life without cheese is no life at all, then don't fret. Enjoy more meatless meals and perhaps later you can tackle cheese—or not. However, with these products and a rainbow of fruits, vegetables, and whole grains, it's never been easier—or more delicious—to eat meat*less* and even cheese-free. You may surprise yourself with what you miss—or don't. Trust me.

Top Ten Surprises about Eating More Meatless Meals

How we eat comes from years or decades of learned and ingrained habits. After eating a certain way for so long, that way—whatever it may be—just feels normal and natural, even if unhealthy, or even if there's a better way. So when we finally do start eating better, or differently, there's a lot we may be surprised by: how certain foods make us feel, new foods we may like (or hate!), how our tastes change, and more. Below is a list of Top Ten Surprises people tend to encounter when they start eating more animal-free fare.

1. "I FEEL LIKE I ACTUALLY HAVE MORE VARIETY IN MY DIET NOW."

I hear this all the time! Purposely eating more meat-free (and dairy-free) foods opens us up to a whole new world of culinary options. Ever heard of nutritional yeast? Likely not. But people who don't eat (or avoid) cheese will often use it to make cheesy sauces, to put on popcorn, and to add to all kinds of recipes. It's got an addictively-nutty flavor and is incredibly good for you (some brands are packed full of vitamin B_{12} for example). What about almond milk? So many people never even think to try it, but love it once they finally do. The same goes for international foods that you may not have thought to try—General Tso's tofu instead of chicken, chana masala instead of lamb curry, and so on.

2. "I HAVE MORE ENERGY THAN EVER BEFORE!"

Eating cleaner, animal-free foods not only opens up a world of culinary options, but opens up our arteries too. Vegan foods have zero cholesterol, so eating those foods helps get more blood to our hearts and brains—giving us more energy. As well, meatless meals tend to be lower in saturated fat and higher in good things, like fiber, than meat-heavy foods. As long as you don't eat a french fry and french bread diet, you'll probably feel better and have more energy than ever before.

3. "AVOIDING CHEESE WAS WAY EASIER THAN I THOUGHT."

Did you know that cheese and other fatty foods create a dopamine-numbing response? "Once you've so dulled your dopamine response, you may subsequently overeat in an effort to achieve the degree of satisfaction experienced previously, which contributes to unhealthy weight gain," according to Dr.

Michael Greger.[18] It's no wonder that many people are surprised that once they stop eating cheese, they don't really miss it. If you want to avoid cheese—or eat less of it—try going one or two months without it. You'll be surprised how your cheesy cravings subside!

4. "I SHOCKED MY DOCTOR AT HOW MUCH MY CHOLESTEROL DROPPED WITHOUT MEDICINE."

Many doctors don't even know that eating an animal-free diet is medically proven to reverse and prevent heart disease without the use of medicine. So though we can surprise ourselves with how much healthier we can become eating that kind of diet, we can also surprise our doctors! This is especially true when it comes to cholesterol, which is completely (and always) absent from vegan foods.

5. "I ACTUALLY ENJOY VEGETABLES NOW!"

In addition to helping us find and appreciate new foods—like tofu and nutritional yeast—we might not have otherwise tried, eating meat-free foods can shine a bright culinary spotlight on the wide world of produce. So many people grew up without a variety of vegetables in their diet. Ever tried kale? Collards? Brussels sprouts? Oyster mushrooms? Avocados? Turnips? Once you start making a point of learning how to prepare these foods to your liking, you may be shocked at how much you enjoy—and even start to crave—them!

6. "THE THOUGHT OF MEAT JUST DOESN'T APPEAL TO ME ANYMORE."

Nearly everyone was raised eating meat—and before we had healthier ways of getting protein, humans ate meat for thousands of years. So liking the taste of meat is deep-rooted in us. Now, we can get the same taste and texture—and the same (or more) protein through plant-based foods. And once we start focusing our diet more on those foods, many of us are surprised that our cravings and even taste for meat disappears entirely.

7. "I NOW ACTUALLY ENJOY COOKING!"

Personally, I like to cook—but a lot of people find it a chore. Though what if we only think it's a *chore* because it's a *bore*? Cooking the same things all

(Continues)

(*Continued*)

the time—chicken nuggets or pasta with meatballs and such—can get old. Many people who start introducing new, meat-free foods into their kitchen find they love the challenge and novelty of preparing and eating new foods—they learn to love cooking!

8. "I SAVE SO MUCH MONEY NOW!"

Eating meatless foods can be lighter on the planet and our bodies, as well as our wallets. Sure, if you only ever eat the most expensive veggie burgers and dairy-free cheeses—or if you only ever shop at the most expensive natural food stores—you may not reap this benefit. But at its heart, plant-based eating is much more affordable. Buy beans and grains in bulk. Shop at mainstream grocers (even Walmart and Target have loads of meatless options). You'll be healthier, more energetic, and have more money to spend on the fun things in life!

9. "PEOPLE ARE SO INTERESTED AND SUPPORTIVE!"

Let's face it: meat-free eating has become super trendy. There are countless people everywhere doing it—whether becoming vegan or vegetarian, doing Meatless Mondays, or just making a point to incorporate more meatless meals into their diets. So there's a lot of support everywhere we turn now. Sure, you may find some naysayers or people who question your choices, but you'll likely be surprised about how positive and inquisitive people are about it (especially if you yourself are positive and friendly about it).

10. "PIZZA WITHOUT CHEESE IS AMAZING."

Perhaps the number-one thing I hear from people new to plant-based eating is how much they enjoy pizza without the cheese! In Italy and throughout the Mediterranean (the home of pizza), cheese is actually used only sparingly on pizzas—it's really only in America that it tends to come slathered in (and even stuffed with) thick dairy. Eating pizza without the cheese, many people find, is actually far more enjoyable. First, because you can usually eat more of it without feeling gross after, and also because the full flavor of the tomato sauce and spices and veggies and crust come through when they're not drowned out by greasy cheese. Give it a shot—you'll be pleasantly surprised!

6

Fill Your Plate: Getting Protein
(and Other Important Nutrients)

Having been a 300-pound NFL linebacker, David Carter is probably one of the last people you'd envision adopting a plant-based diet. It took him by surprise, too. The grandson of a Los Angeles barbeque restaurateur, Carter spent his youth eating mounds of chicken, beef, and pork.

His dream from the time he was young was to be a professional football player. With his cousins and brother, he'd play football in the streets of his South Central L.A. neighborhood after school every day with a laser focus. He eventually played for UCLA, the Arizona Cardinals, Oakland Raiders, Jacksonville Jaguars, Dallas Cowboys, and the Chicago Bears.

Being a football player reinforced Carter's belief that he needed to eat meat—and lots of it—to be big and strong.

"Every coach, trainer, nutritionist, and doctor all pointed me in the direction of animal products," says Carter. "From protein shakes to weight gainers there was no other alternative, so I did as I was told and followed the standard athlete's diet regimen. Whey protein, raw eggs, gallons of milk, and casein were in just about every supplement I took."[1]

Carter's wife, Paige, became vegetarian and later vegan. Though Carter admired her conviction to eat in line with her values, he also thought it was something he could personally never do while playing football.

But all that changed after watching the film *Forks Over Knives*. He had been suffering from nagging injuries—tendinitis, arthritis, and muscle fatigue. He'd also read that the average life expectancy of a football player is in the mid- to late-fifties, two decades shorter than that of the average male.[2] While there have been conflicting studies on this topic, defensive linemen, in particular Carter's position, were singled out by the National Institute for Occupational Safety and Health as having a 50 percent greater risk of death from heart disease than the general population.[3]

"I learned the consumption of meat, eggs, and dairy are directly linked to the top killers of Americans," says Carter, after watching *Forks Over Knives*. "The very things we've been hearing since we were kids that do our bodies good are clogging our arteries, giving us diabetes, making us obese, and are putting the current generation of kids on the path toward a host of chronic, preventable diseases that will end up shortening their lives and causing untold suffering."[4] Carter's Valentine's Day gift to his wife that year: adopting a plant-based diet.

Carter saw performance benefits quickly. His small injuries and muscle fatigue disappeared, and his recovery time and endurance improved, enabling him to train even harder.

Carter needs to consume 10,000 calories daily to keep weight on while training. He eats up to six meals a day, fueling up with nutrient-dense meals such as beans and rice with vegetables or sprouted grains with legumes. And what about protein?

"I'm a 300-plus-pound vegan; I'm living proof you don't have to kill animals to gain muscle," he said.[5]

So Where Do You Get Your Protein?

Our society is protein-obsessed. Ask any vegetarian or vegan the most common question they're asked, and it's bound to be, "Where do you get your protein?"

But that's slowly changing, as Carter and a long list of pro athletes—including tennis legends Venus Williams and Martina Navratilova, Olympic gold medalist Carl Lewis, quarterback Joe Namath,

MMA fighter Mac Danzig, Ironman triathlete Brendan Brazier, ultra-marathoner Rich Roll, and bodybuilder Robert Cheeke, to name a handful—expound publicly on how their athletic performance has been enhanced by eating plant-based diets.

Although we're talking about *reducing* meat consumption, you may opt to embrace a vegetarian or vegan diet. So let's tackle some of the most pernicious nutrition myths about eating plant-based. Below, I've outlined some of the properties of the most common nutrients people associate with meat; for more detailed information on nutrients in a plant-based diet, check out *Vegan for Life:*

> **Did you know?**
>
> The average woman needs about 46 grams of protein each day, and the average man needs 56 grams.[6] Even vegetarians and vegans consume 70 percent more protein than they need every day.[7]

Everything You Need to Know to Be Healthy and Fit on a Plant-Based Diet by dietitians Jack Norris and Virginia Messina. Or check out their websites, jacknorrisrd.com and theveganrd.com.

Protein

Although vegetarians' and vegans' protein intake seems to be one of the top concerns of their meat-eating friends and relatives, it's actually one of the nutrients of least medical concern. According to Dr. Michael Greger, less than 3 percent of Americans are protein deficient, presumably because they're simply not eating enough food in general.[8]

"Vegetarians and vegans get 70 percent more protein than they need every day," according to Greger.

Of course it's true that we need protein to be healthy, but what's protein, anyway? And what does it do? Proteins are molecules made up of smaller building blocks of molecules called amino acids. Twenty different amino acids combine to make the various proteins we need. Our bodies create some amino acids and can modify some others.[9] We must consume some of those essential amino acids in our food.[10] We use protein in order to make hormones, enzymes, and other chemicals as well as to create skin, muscles, bones, cartilage, and the hemoglobin in our blood.[11]

As the Harvard School of Public Health explains, "Protein is found throughout the body—in muscle, bone, skin, hair, and virtually every other body part or tissue. It makes up the enzymes that power many chemical reactions and the hemoglobin that carries oxygen in your blood. At least ten thousand different proteins make you what you are and keep you that way."[12]

Although how they get protein is a common question for vegans and vegetarians, protein is actually found in abundance in plant-based foods. You can consume it in the form of nuts and in beans—black beans, pinto beans, garbanzo beans (chickpeas), or kidney beans. Spreads such as hummus and peanut or almond butter are great sources of protein, as are lentils and split peas. Seeds are also high in protein, especially sunflower, hemp, chia, and pumpkin.

Another protein-packed seed—quinoa—is taking the United States by storm. In 2004, the *Wall Street Journal* reported, "US imports of quinoa—grown mainly in the Andes Mountains of South America— soared to 68.9 million pounds last year from 7.66 million pounds in 2007, according to trade-data provider Datamyne Inc."[13] This popular superfood packs a powerful protein punch of 8 grams of protein per cooked cup.

Of course there's soy protein in tofu, tempeh, soy milk, and plant-based meats such as veggie dogs, burgers, and nuggets.[14] All of these plant foods are excellent sources of protein that will help your body perform its essential functions and help you feel full.

And check out the tables below for some surprising facts on protein content of some popular plant-based foods. Perhaps the biggest surprises of all are that we don't need as much protein as we think, and many vegetables are good sources of protein. When you consider the average woman needs about 46 grams of protein per day and the average man needs about 56, you'll see that we can easily meet that need with meatless foods.[15]

Table 6.1 Protein in Common Plant Foods

FOOD	SERVING SIZE	AMOUNT OF PROTEIN
Cooked black beans	½ cup	8 grams
Cooked pinto beans	½ cup	8 grams
Cooked garbanzo beans	½ cup	8 grams
Smooth peanut butter	2 tablespoons	8 grams
Almond butter	2 tablespoons	6.7 grams
Hummus	½ cup	7.8 grams
Shelled sunflower seeds	¼ cup	6.4 grams
Hemp seeds	3 tablespoons	10 grams
Chia seeds	2 tablespoons	6 grams
Pumpkin seeds	¼ cup, roasted without salt	17 grams
Quinoa	1 cup, cooked	8.1 grams
Tofu	3 ounces	8 grams
Tempeh	3 ounces	16 grams
Soy milk	1 cup	7 grams
Edamame	½ cup	11 grams
Beyond Meat Beefy Crumbles	½ cup	13 grams
Beyond Chicken Southwest Style Strips	6 strips	20 grams

Sources: Beltsville Human Nutrition Research Center, Beyondmeat.com, Bob's Red Mill, Soyfoods Association of North America, US Department of Agriculture, and Wolfram Alpha Computational Knowledge Engine.

As you can see, there are ample plant-based sources of protein that, when stacked up throughout the day, enable you to meet or well exceed your recommended daily intake. Here are some comparable animal-based foods, including a couple chicken entrees, that people tend to think of as healthier food. As the charts illustrate, these tend to be higher in calories and fat and have little fiber.

Table 6.2 Calories, Fat, Protein, and Fiber in a Few Common Plant-Based Foods

PLANT-STRONG PROTEIN	CALORIES	TOTAL FAT (GRAMS)	PROTEIN (GRAMS)	FIBER (GRAMS)
Vegetable lentil soup (1 can)	320	4	18	10
Veggie dog	50	2	7	1
Peanut butter and pumpkin spread sandwich	350	18	12	6
Beefless burger, plain	243	7	20	3.5
Bean & rice burrito with salsa	368	5.5	15	14

Sources: Lightlife.com, Progresso.com, and USDA National Nutrient Database for Standard Reference.

Table 6.3 Calories, Fat, Protein, and Fiber in a Few Common Animal-Based Foods

ANIMAL PROTEIN	CALORIES	TOTAL FAT (GRAMS)	PROTEIN (GRAMS)	FIBER (GRAMS)
Chicken corn chowder (1 can)	400	18	14	4
Hot dog	170	15	6	0
Sausage biscuit, fast food style	420	27	11	0.5
Hamburger, fast food style, plain	232	9	13	1
Chicken pot pie, frozen entree	616	36	15	3
Fast food chicken salad cup	360	24	28	2
Fast food shredded chicken burrito	400	18	16	3

Sources: Chick-fil-A, Kraftrecipes.com, Progresso.com, Tacobell.com, and USDA National Nutrient Database for Standard Reference.

Iron

Iron is an essential mineral that helps our muscles use and store oxygen, transport oxygen through our bodies, and, as a component of enzymes, helps us digest our food, among other things—and it's found in abundance in plant foods.[16] Everyone should make sure to get enough of this vital mineral.

Table 6.4 Iron in Common Foods

Recommended dietary allowance for adults/day: male, 8 mg; female, 18 mg.

FOOD	SERVING SIZE	NUTRIENT CONTENT
Quick oats, dry	1 cup	29.9 mg
Spinach, cooked	1 cup	6.4 mg
Canned tomato sauce	1 cup	2.5 mg
Roasted chicken	1 cup	1.69 mg
Steak	3 ounces	1.5 mg
Hard-boiled egg	1	1.62 mg

Sources: Oregon State University Nutrient Information Center and USDA Nutrient List.

Table 6.5 Best Plant-Based Sources of Iron

FOOD	SERVING SIZE	AMOUNT OF IRON
Canned white beans	1 cup	3 mg
Cooked lentils	1 cup	6 mg
Boiled spinach	1 cup	6.4 mg
Canned kidney beans	1 cup	5 mg
Canned chickpeas	1 cup	5 mg
Prune juice	1 cup	3 mg
Roasted pumpkin seeds	4 tablespoons	5 mg

Sources: National Institutes of Health, Oregon State University Nutrient Information Center, USDA Dietary Guidelines for Americans 2005.

Although registered dietitian Jack Norris says, "You do not need to worry about iron if you are otherwise healthy and eat a varied vegetarian or vegan diet," Norris and *Vegan for Life* co-author Virginia Messina, RD, suggest that if you're getting all your dietary iron from plant sources, it's helpful to use strategies to boost absorption.[17] The most effective way is to add vitamin C to meals. This can be done by enjoying a glass of orange juice with your meal, or eating broccoli; yellow, green, or red peppers; green leafy vegetables such as kale, collards, and Swiss chard; Brussels sprouts; cauliflower; and strawberries.[18] "The effects of vitamin C on iron absorption are rather dramatic," they say.[19]

Vitamin B$_{12}$

It's important to note that there's one vitamin unavailable from plant sources: vitamin B$_{12}$, which is essential for nervous system function, DNA synthesis, and proper red blood cell formation.[20]

Fortunately, B$_{12}$ is produced by bacteria or microbes and thus doesn't require an animal source.[21] The bacteria grow in the intestines of animals, which is why meat and animal products can be a source of vitamin B$_{12}$. Although we may have once been able to obtain B$_{12}$ from natural sources, in developed countries we chlorinate water and kill off any microbes, so now we need to obtain it from other sources.[22]

For those switching to an entirely plant-based or vegan diet (and frankly, for anyone, since many people who eat meat are often still B$_{12}$ deficient), Dr. Michael Greger recommends supplementing, especially if you're a woman who's pregnant or nursing. Fortunately it's easy to obtain all the B$_{12}$ we need in fortified foods *and* supplements.[23] Of course anyone making major diet changes should talk with a physician or dietitian knowledgeable about plant-based diets.

According to Dr. Greger, "The cheapest way to get our B$_{12}$ is probably with one 2,500 microgram sublingual, chewable, or liquid supplement of cyanocobalamin once a week. The stuff is dirt cheap. You can find a twenty-year supply online for $40. All the B$_{12}$ our body needs for $2 a year! Of course, the stuff doesn't last twenty years. It has a four-year expiration date, so share it with some friends."[24] Other foods fortified with B$_{12}$ include some (but not all) soy milks, plant-based meats (meat-free burgers, etc.), nutritional yeast (more on this veg staple later, see page 124), and energy bars.[25]

Calcium

The *Got Milk?* ad campaign had many of us believing milk was synonymous with calcium. The dairy industry is in schools, giving out free posters, lesson plans, funds for promoting dairy, and in some instances even bringing a cow to school, all to try to persuade American children to believe that we need milk for strong bones.[27] By the time we're old enough to think for ourselves, we're terrified that we'll get osteoporosis if we don't chug glasses of milk every day, pour it all over our cereal, and pile cheese high on our plates.

The reality is there are many sources of calcium that are better for us because they don't come with the saturated fat and cholesterol inherent in dairy milk. (In fact, cheese, pizza, and ice cream are the biggest sources of saturated fat in Americans' diets.[28])

But here's the deal: lactose intolerance is prevalent among Americans, with researchers from Cornell University reporting an estimated 30 to 50 million Americans are lactose intolerant. It's especially common among non-whites with as many as 75 percent of African Americans and American Indians and 90 percent of Asian Americans being lactose intolerant. Those who are lactose intolerant often experience bloating, cramping, nausea, gas, and diarrhea after consuming foods or beverages containing the milk sugar lactose.[29] Lactose intolerance actually makes sense: humans are the only species of animal that drinks the milk of another species, and that drinks milk after infancy. Adult humans are simply not evolved to drink milk. Milk also is one of the most typical food allergens, according to the American College of Allergy, Asthma & Immunology, particularly among children. Dairy allergies may result in an upset stomach, vomiting, bloody stools, and even anaphylactic shock.[30]

> **Did you know?**
>
> Greens are a great source of calcium. One cup of cooked collards contains 357 mg of calcium, while 1 cup of nonfat milk contains 299 mg.[26]

Table 6.6 Calcium in Common Foods

Recommended dietary allowance for adults/day: male, 1,000 mg; female: 1,000 mg

FOOD	SERVING SIZE	NUTRIENT CONTENT
Firm tofu	1 cup	507 mg
White beans	1 cup	93 mg
Collards	1 cup	268 mg
Orange juice, added calcium	1 cup	347 mg
American cheese	1 cup	598 mg
Nonfat milk with added vitamins A and D	1 cup	299 mg
Sesame seeds	3.5 ounces	975 mg

Sources: Oregon State University Nutrient Information Center and USDA Nutrient List.

Table 6.7 Best Plant-Based Sources of Calcium

FOOD	SERVING SIZE	AMOUNT OF CALCIUM
Canned white beans	1 cup	93 mg
Cooked bok choy	1 cup	141 mg
Dried figs	1 cup	181 mg
Orange	1 medium	60 mg
Almonds	¼ cup	100 mg
Firm tofu	1 cup	507 mg
Turnip greens	1 cup	216 mg

Sources: National Institutes of Health and Oregon State University Nutrient Information Center.

The great news is there are plenty of sources of calcium that don't involve cows. Leafy green vegetables—collard greens, kale, Swiss chard, turnip and mustard greens, and spinach—are some great calcium-loaded greens.[31] Other sources include lentils, tofu, broccoli, almonds, bok choy, and even sesame seeds—and these are just to name a few. To top it off, you get something not found in milk when you get your calcium from these sources: fiber and antioxidants, and you don't get the saturated fat, cholesterol, antibiotics, and hormones that may be in cows' milk.[32]

Omega-3s

Omega-3 fatty acids have been the subject of much attention, with good reason. They contribute to a number of our bodily functions, including helping with blood clotting. They are also associated with numerous health benefits such as protection against some of the top killers of Americans: heart disease, cancer, and stroke.[33] Unfortunately, omega-3 deficiency is common among Americans—whether omnivorous, plant-based, or somewhere in between.

There are three types of omega-3s in our diets: alpha-linolenic acid (ALA), eicosapentaenoic acid (EPA), and docosahexaenoic acid (DHA).[34] ALA can be found in canola and soybean oils, flaxseeds and flaxseed oil, in walnuts, some green vegetables, such as kale, spinach, salad greens, and Brussels sprouts. EPA and DHA can be partially converted by our bodies from ALA.[35] Although fish is an often recommended source of omega-3s, it sometimes comes with undesirable accompaniments: mercury, PCBs, and dioxin, toxins that may actually increase our risk of the very things omega-3s can help prevent: cancer, cardiac death, and type 2 diabetes.[36]

Fortunately, there are plant-based sources of DHA and EPA that are derived from microalgae, the same source from which fish get their omega-3s.[37] The plant-based sources, however, are grown in a sanitary lab environment, eliminating the need for concern about ocean-borne toxins found in their fish-based counterparts like fish oil.[38]

A 2015 *Washington Post* article wrote of fish oil, "The vast majority of research published recently in major journals provides no evidence of a health benefit. . . . Andrew Grey and Mark Bolland, researchers at the University of Auckland in New Zealand, for example, reviewed fish oil research published in major journals between 2005 and 2012 based on randomized clinical trials; twenty-two of the 24 studies showed no benefit, according to their work published in *JAMA Internal Medicine*."[39]

Table 6.8 Omega-3 Fatty Acids in Common Foods

Adequate intake for adults/day: male, 1.6 g; female, 1.1 g

FOOD	SERVING SIZE	NUTRIENT CONTENT
Flaxseed oil	1 tablespoon	7.3 g (ALA)
Chia seeds	1 ounce	5.1 g (ALA)
Walnuts	1 ounce	2.6 g (ALA)
Tuna, canned, white	3 ounces	.74 g (EPA+DHA)
Atlantic salmon	3 ounces	1.23 g (EPA+DHA)
Navy beans	1 cup	1.1 g (ALA)
Pacific herring	3 ounces	1.8 g (EPA+DHA)

Source: Oregon State University Nutrient Information Center.

Table 6.9 Best Plant-Based Sources of Omega-3s

FOOD	SERVING SIZE	AMOUNT OF OMEGA 3
Chia seeds	1 ounce	5.1 g (ALA)
Flaxseeds	1 ounce	6.3 g (ALA)
Walnuts	1 ounce	2.6 g (ALA)

Source: DHA-EPA Omega-3 Institute.

No matter what your diet, you might want to consider one of the algae-based supplements. You might also want to try eating at least one source of omega-3s daily, that is, ground flaxseed in a smoothie, chia seeds, hemp seeds (for more on these, see the special ingredients section on page 124), or flaxseed or walnuts in your breakfast cereal, or atop salad, or flax oil as a dressing.[40]

Striking the Right Balance

Of course, it's easy for us to obsess over single nutrients. Though none of us should take this lightly in order to ensure we're getting our essential vitamins and minerals, it's easy to be healthy with a varied, balanced, plant-based diet—it really is that straightforward. Don't let the notion of nutrients make meat*less* seem daunting. Whether you're going meatless on Mondays, flexing your diet, or jumping into eating solely plant-based foods, be sure that you're enjoying a wide array of fruits, vegetables, whole grains, nuts, seeds, and legumes. Not only will the rainbow of colors of fruits and vegetables help you get all the important nutrients your body needs, it will also prevent you from getting bored with what you're eating. And if you're looking for suggestions, the recipes in Chapter 8 are a great place to start.

PART III

Recipes for Success

7

Vegetable Stock:
Ingredients, Shopping, Swaps,
and Other Basics

While there are many great reasons to eat meatless—like feeling and looking better, helping animals, and improving the health of the planet—many people will say the best part is the food itself!

Of course, making any shift in how you eat can be daunting, especially if you're not used to cooking. The good news is that, even if you can't boil water, or if you're a regular Julia Child, it's easy to eat meatless at home.

Here are some tips for what to look for in the grocery store and simple swaps to make meal prep easy, followed by a few of my favorite combos.

Grocery Shopping

Although many foods we eat are already meat free (produce, pastas, breads, grains, and so much more), here are some foods you might be unfamiliar with as well as information on where to find them. New products are being developed all the time; these are some popular brands at the time of writing.

Proteins

Veggie burgers are an easy option to have on hand for a quick, yet filling meal. From more meat-like burgers to more vegetable-filled grain burgers there are dozens of varieties, so sample them until you find your favorites.

Beefy crumbles make simple substitutions for ground beef and chorizo in tacos, spaghetti, and shepherd's pie. These are family favorites that can be ready in minutes.

From breakfast patties to maple breakfast links to Italian links and beer brats, you can find meatless versions of any **sausage** in the refrigerator section of most stores.

Seitan is a hearty meatless meat that's an excellent source of protein, made from gluten, the protein of wheat. It can be purchased in strips or loaves and is delicious barbecued, stir fried, marinated and grilled, and more. If you love cooking, try making your own. You can freeze it to have plenty on hand.

Tempeh is a fermented soy-based protein. It's perfect for sandwiches, marinated and cooked as bacon, and sautéed in entrees.

Tofu is a versatile protein from Asia that has been eaten for thousands of years. Firm tofu can be baked, stir-fried, deep fried, and used as a center-of-plate protein, a salad topping, and more. Soft (or silken) tofu can be used in baking and desserts.

Animal-Free Dairy

Try dairy-free **margarines**, such as Earth Balance, Smart Balance, and Miyoko's European Style Cultured VeganButter.

Dairy-free **cream cheeses**—those made by Tofutti, Kite Hill, and Follow Your Heart—are excellent for smearing on bagels or baked into a cheesecake. Even Trader Joe's has a store-brand dairy-free cream cheese!

Instead of dairy milk, try **soy, almond, or coconut milk**—sample all of them until you find one you like.

Dairy-free **yogurts** are available in abundance, made from soy, almond, and coconut milk and available from brands like Silk, So Delicious, Stonyfield, Kite Hill, Daiya, and Trader Joe's.

Condiments

Spreads like Just Mayo, Vegenaise, and Mindful Mayo make creamy sandwich spreads and are excellent ingredients for sauces and dips.

In the Freezer

Proteins

Edamame (soybeans in the pod) are delicious high-protein snacks or appetizers when boiled and salted in the shell. Shelled, they make a wonderful addition to stir fry recipes and salads, adding vibrant color and a nutty flavor.

You can find a variety of **veggie burgers** in the freezer section as well. Gardein, Beyond Meat, and Boca offer meaty burgers, while Amy's and Dr. Praeger's have grain and vegetable burgers. These burgers are all perfect for the grill!

Meet your **meatless meatballs** in the freezer section from Beyond Meat, and pick up some Gardein Chick'n Scallopini, sweet and sour porkless bites, and beefless tips while you're there. These meaty, protein-packed foods are an easy swap in spaghetti and meatballs, sweet and sour pork, beef with broccoli, or chicken Marsala.

Heat and enjoy **crispy, chicken-free tenders** and **crabless cakes** from Gardein, pockets stuffed with meatless ham and cheese or cheese and pepperoni from Tofurky, or pizzas from Daiya and Amy's. These options make easy weeknight meals when you don't feel like cooking.

Speaking of Amy's, the company offers a wide range of **frozen meals** from sides of mac and cheese to entrees of noodle stir fry, baked ziti bowl, pad Thai, burritos, breakfast bowls, and more.

Ice Cream

Most grocery stores now carry dairy-free ice creams. So Delicious makes a variety of mouth-watering flavors. Tofutti is a classic, and Trader Joe's offers its own brand. And, drumroll . . . in 2016, Ben & Jerry's rolled out vegan versions of classics Chunky Monkey, Chocolate Fudge Brownie, Coffee Caramel Fudge, and PB & Cookies—all made with creamy, delicious almond milk instead of cows' milk.

Grains

You can purchase frozen brown rice, steel-cut oats, and other grains to make eating healthy super simple. Just reheat in the microwave for a minute when you're ready to eat.

On the Shelf (Non-Perishable Items)
Grains, Seeds, Spices, and Dry Goods

Though **white rice** is certainly vegan and yummy, **brown rice** is more nutritious and has a nutty flavor and chewy texture.

Steel-cut oats (the inner kernel of whole oats) make for hearty breakfasts, and many people may not realize they're also an inexpensive meat replacement, when cooked al dente, in chili and tacos. You can now even find quick-cooking steel-cut oats that can be ready in fewer than five minutes.

Did you know?

Peas and lentils run at about 7 cents for a ½ cup serving compared to 67 and 71 cents, and $1.07 for a 3-ounce serving of chicken, pork, and beef, respectively.[1]

Flax meal (ground flax seeds) can replace eggs in baked goods. Simply combine 1 tablespoon flax meal with 2 tablespoons water, stir vigorously, and add to mixture.

Powdered egg replacers such as Ener-G egg replacer make easy alternatives to eggs in cookies, cakes, and breads.

Know how to boil water? Then you can make **quinoa**. It's protein rich and quick to prepare. Purchase it in bulk or in a box. Boil water, add the grain, and cook for 15 minutes, then fluff. Ta da! Some varieties are pre-rinsed. If not, it's advised to rinse to avoid a bitter flavor.

Seeds like **chia**, **flax**, and **pumpkin** are good sources of protein, omega-3 fatty acids, and essential minerals. You can usually find these seeds with other nuts and more commonly known seeds. They all make excellent toppings for salads and cereals. Chia seeds can make a delicious, easy breakfast pudding when combined with almond milk, sweetener, and fruit.

Barley, buckwheat, millet, and **farro** are all whole grains and make excellent alternatives to rice or noodles to add variety. They can be cooked with broth and herbs for a delicious pilaf or boiled and strained to top a salad.

Nut butters—peanut, almond, and sunflower—are a delicious and easy way to add protein to smoothies, on a sandwich, of course, or on toast with a banana, for a stick to your ribs breakfast.

Vegetable bouillon or broth is a key ingredient to keep in the cupboard for soup bases, sauces, gravies, and more.

Vegetable shortening is useful in baking biscuits and scones. I get the nonhydrogenated variety, such as the Spectrum brand, to avoid trans fats.

Soy sauce, tamari, and **Bragg's Liquid Aminos** are all condiments and typically found with Asian foods. They can add a salty flavor to gravies and Asian-inspired sauces.

Liquid smoke adds a hickory flavor to foods such as chilis and soup. Use it in extreme moderation, as it can be overpowering.

Nori flakes can be found in the international section of some supermarkets or in Asian markets. They're flaked bits of nori, the seaweed we're most familiar with, to make sushi. They add a hint of sea flavoring. If you can't find nori flakes, you can make your own by crumbling or tearing up a sheet of nori.

Beans

Beans and legumes are excellent and inexpensive protein sources and there's a huge variety: chickpeas, pinto beans, black beans, kidney beans, cannellini beans, black eyed peas, split peas, and many, many more. Lentils are one of the cheapest sources of protein and can cook in just minutes. You can get red lentils, black lentils, and French green lentils. Canned beans are slightly more costly yet still far less expensive than meat. As a bonus, you can use the juice from your can of beans as an egg replacer. I haven't lost my mind. Look up "aquafaba" online.

Build a Bowl

Bowls have quickly become a popular meal, and restaurant chains that specialize in a variety of them have been popping up around the country. Bowls range from the super simple to fancy schmancy. At home, they can be simple, filling, cheap, nutritious, and easy to assemble for a weeknight meal. Here are some favorites for inspiration. Keep in mind there are no rules.

The basic formula is this: big bowl + grain base (rice, quinoa, barley, millet, noodles, etc.) + protein (beans, legumes, tofu, tempeh, or seitan, for example) + vegetables (broccoli, carrots, cabbage, squash, peas, you get the picture) + sauce (soy sauce plus sriracha, peanut sauce, cashew cream, miso tahini, pesto, and so on). Yes, it's that easy and, no, you can't mess this up! Here are some fun bowls you can make at home.

Mexican Fiesta Bowl
Base: white rice, brown rice, or both
Protein: beans (black, pinto, whatever you like)
Veggies: chopped tomato, shredded lettuce, avocado, cilantro
Sauce: salsa or guacamole
Bonus: tortilla strips

Japanese Noodle Bowl

Base: udon or soba noodles
Protein: edamame or baked tofu
Veggies: shredded cabbage, carrots, onions
Sauce: teriyaki sauce or a mix of soy sauce, garlic, sriracha, ginger, and sesame oil
Bonus: sesame seeds

Baked Potato Bowl

Base: sweet or white potato, baked
Protein: Twenty-minute two bean chili (see page 188)
Veggies: broccoli florets, or chives or green onions
Sauce: cheese sauce from Macaroni and Cashew Cheese Surprise recipe (see page 189)
Bonus: dollop of dairy-free sour cream

Indonesian Peanut Bowl

Base: soba noodles or spaghetti
Protein: peanuts
Veggies: carrots, snow peas, cabbage, broccoli
Sauce: peanut sauce from Noodles with Peanut Sauce recipe (see page 185)
Bonus: red chili flakes

Italian Bowl

Base: angel hair or spaghetti
Protein: cannellini beans
Veggies: broccoli, asparagus, artichokes, olives
Sauce: pesto (see page 180) or marinara
Bonus: sliced meatless Italian sausages

Sushi Bowl

Base: brown or white rice
Protein: edamame or tofu
Veggies: avocado, carrots, cucumbers, asparagus
Sauce: soy sauce or tamari
Bonus: nori flakes

Indian Bowl

Base: brown rice, basmati rice, quinoa
Protein: chickpeas or red lentils
Veggies: cauliflower, green beans, eggplant
Sauce: red curry paste blended with coconut milk
Bonus: papadum (Indian crackers)

Mediterranean Bowl

Base: couscous, bulgur, barley
Protein: chickpeas, hummus, falafel
Veggies: cucumbers, tomatoes, olives, red onions
Sauce: miso tahini from Vitality Bowl recipe (see page 176)
    or plain, unsweetened, dairy-free yogurt
Bonus: pita wedges

Creole Bowl

Base: brown or white rice
Protein: red beans
Veggies: okra, tomatoes, bell peppers
Sauce: Tabasco or Crystal hot sauce
Bonus: cornbread

Hawaiian Bowl

Base: brown or white rice
Protein: baked tofu, tempeh, cashews
Veggies: red and green peppers, zucchini
Sauce: teriyaki
Bonus: pineapple

Simple Swaps

Agood first step is to consider some of your favorite dishes and how to make them meatless. If it's hard to come up with ideas, track what you eat for a week so you can record what you typically eat. At the end of the week, go over the list and consider what things will be easiest to change. For some dishes, it may be as easy as leaving out the meat or replacing it with a vegetarian meat. Others may require a little more work.

INSTEAD OF	TRY
Beef in tacos, enchiladas, and burritos	Lentils, pinto, or black beans
Cows' milk	Almond, soy, or coconut milk
Grilled chicken skewers	Beyond Chicken and vegetable skewers
Butter	Dairy-free butter or margarine
Pasta with meatballs	Pasta primavera or meatless meatballs
Eggs in baking	Flax meal, mashed banana, or Ener-G egg replacer
Chicken nuggets	Meatless chicken tenders
Scrambled eggs	Tofu or chickpea scramble

What the Heck Are Flaxseeds
(and a Few Other Unusual Ingredients)?

By now you probably realize eating meatless can be a cinch. Although it's not necessary to fill your cupboards with new-to-you foods, some people find eating meatless opens up a fresh world of food. Here are a few foods that add variety, flavor, and nutrients to a plant-based diet:

Chia seeds: Yep, the same seeds that provided wooly sprouts to our ceramic pets have become superfoods, leading us to wonder why we wasted them as a decoration for so long. Rich in omega-3s, calcium, antioxidants, and fiber, the seeds can add nutrients in cereals, smoothies, desserts, and atop salads.[2] With some oats, mashed bananas, and soy or almond milk, they make a great "overnight oats"—a quick, healthy breakfast.

Flaxseeds: Small golden or brown seeds are often ground into a flour to create flax meal. These seeds have been named "one of the most powerful foods on the planet" and hailed as a super food for their nutritional benefits. Those benefits include being rich in lignans and omega-3s, protein, fiber, B vitamins, and more.[3] If consumed whole, you may not digest them and receive those nutritional benefits, so it's best to buy them ground or grind them at home in a coffee grinder. Sprinkle atop salads and soups for a nutty flavor, add them to pancakes, waffles, and smoothies for a nutrient boost, or use them as an egg replacer in baked goods.

Hemp seeds: These seeds from the cannabis plant are in the same family as marijuana, but don't worry; they won't get you high. However, they will give you a nutritional boost. They're small, fine seeds that are a protein powerhouse and are loaded with omega-3s and essential amino acids. You can sprinkle them on top of salads and cereals and put them in smoothies—maybe you're detecting a theme here. Use them instead of breadcrumbs to coat tofu or seitan to add flavor and nutrients.[4]

Nutritional yeast is available as a powder or as flakes. It has a flavor some call nutty, some call cheesy, and I call delicious. Nutritional yeast is deactivated yeast made from molasses.[5] It's high in protein, low in calories, and some brands—not all—are fortified with vitamin B_{12}. It can be sprinkled atop toast, bagels, baked potatoes, or popcorn, and used in gravies or sauces to add flavor. One of my favorite applications is combined with cashews and soy milk to make cheese for macaroni and cheese or nacho cheese (see recipe page 189).

Miso paste is fermented soybean paste that adds a salty, umami flavor to dishes. It's delicious in gravies, sauces, creams, and, of course, it is the key ingredient in fast, delicious traditional Japanese miso soup.

Texturized vegetable protein (TVP): this old-school vegetarian meat replacer found in health food stores provides an inexpensive, toothsome texture to chili, spaghetti sauce, or soup. It has to be rehydrated before use and will soak up the flavors of the foods it's applied to.

Corn flour is finely ground cornmeal, perfect for baking cornbread, muffins, or cornmeal pancakes. It's different from cornstarch. Using cornstarch in these applications wouldn't turn out so great.

Tahini is a paste made from sesame seeds and is a standard ingredient in Middle Eastern recipes and excellent for sauces and spreads.

Agave is a liquid sweetener made from an agave plant—the same plant from which tequila is made. Some people like to use it in place of sugar or honey in beverages or on top of cereal.

8

Recipes for Success

Many of these easy recipes are some I make at home that my family loves. I hope you'll enjoy them too. Chef Alex Bury, who I introduced in Chapter 5, shares many of her favorites as well. Most are easy enough for someone who's new to the kitchen and plant-based cooking. A few require some additional steps and ingredients that may be new to you. Have fun and enjoy the process!

Breakfast

Very Berry Scones

These crumbly, yet soft scones are perfect for impressing friends with a fancy brunch or tea party, or a bring-along breakfast for a road trip. The lemon complements the berries adding a hint of citrus. You can freeze the dough and bake later for a quick, decadent weekday breakfast.

MAKES 6 to 8
TIME: 35 minutes; 15 minutes active

1 cup white flour
1 cup whole wheat flour
¼ cup sugar
2 teaspoons baking powder
¼ teaspoon salt
⅓ cup dairy-free margarine, such as Earth Balance

¾ cup plain, unsweetened soy or almond milk
1 teaspoon vanilla or lemon extract
1 teaspoon lemon zest
1 cup mixed berries, fresh or frozen

Preheat oven to 400°F.

If using frozen berries, thaw them in warm water and strain well.

In a large bowl, mix together both flours, sugar, baking powder, and salt. Separate margarine into 6 pieces and add to the flour mixture using a fork or pastry cutter to cut in until the margarine is evenly distributed, with no pieces larger than a pea.

Combine the soy or almond milk, vanilla or lemon extract, and zest and pour this into the dry mixture. Stir until the dough comes together. Add berries and gently fold into the dough. Some berries may get squashed and add a hint of purple—that's okay.

Once the dough is thoroughly mixed with the berries, place it on a lightly floured surface and flatten to about ¾ of an inch thick. Using a biscuit cutter or the mouth of a tumbler, cut the dough into 6 or 8 scones. You may need to reform the dough into a ball and press it out again to make all the scones. Place on an ungreased baking sheet. Sprinkle tops with additional sugar, optionally. Bake for 20 minutes, until tops are golden brown.

> **PRO-TIP:** You can substitute berries with your favorite fruit. Or go crazy and use chocolate chips. If you do that, use the vanilla extract rather than the lemon.

To freeze: Shape the scones per instructions, place on a baking sheet, cover with plastic wrap, and put in the freezer. Once they've set long enough to hold their shape—about 4 hours to overnight—place into freezer bags or containers and store in the freezer until you're ready to eat them, up to a couple of months. When you're ready to eat them, remove from the freezer and place on baking sheets while the oven is preheating. Bake as per instructions, adding an extra 2 minutes if necessary to reach golden brown.

Banana Walnut Pancakes

With flavors reminiscent of a warm, fresh loaf of banana bread, these fluffy pancakes are as easy as they are delicious. Top with warm maple syrup and sprinkle with more bananas and nuts for a filling breakfast.

MAKES 6 to 8 pancakes
TIME: 20 minutes active

1 cup whole wheat or white flour, or a combination of the two
1 tablespoon granulated sugar or agave nectar
2 tablespoons baking powder
⅛ teaspoon salt

1 banana, mashed
¼ cup walnut pieces
1 cup plain, unsweetened soy or almond milk, ¼ cup more if you like thinner pancakes

Combine the flour, sugar (if using), baking powder, and salt in a bowl and mix. Add the banana and walnuts, and mix. Add soy milk (add agave here, if using that instead of sugar) and beat until the batter is fully mixed. If you like thinner pancakes, you can add another ¼ cup of milk or even water.

Warm a nonstick skillet on medium-high. Measure about ⅓ cup of the batter onto the warm skillet. When bubbles start to appear on the top, after about 2 to 3 minutes, flip. Let brown for about 2 minutes and re move from heat, and repeat. Keep cooked pancakes warm by placing on a plate and covering with a clean dishtowel or in an oven at 200°F until all the pancakes are cooked. Serve with your favorite syrup or fruit topping.

Tropical Pancakes

Top your pancakes off with pineapple and coconut and enjoy with a side of mango, bananas, or your favorite fruit for a visit to the tropics on a Sunday morning.

MAKES 6 to 8
TIME: 20 minutes active

1 cup whole wheat or white flour, or a combination of the two
1 tablespoon sugar or agave nectar
2 tablespoons baking powder
⅛ teaspoon salt
¼ cup flaked coconut plus more for garnish
½ cup plain, unsweetened soy or almond milk

½ cup pineapple juice or additional soy or almond milk (you can use the juice that was in the can with the pineapple rings if using)
2 tablespoons vegetable oil
1 8-ounce can pineapple rings or pineapple preserves

Combine the flour, sugar (if using), baking powder, salt, and coconut in a bowl and mix. Add the milk, pineapple juice, agave (if using), and oil, and beat until the batter is smooth. If you like a thinner pancake, you can add another ¼ cup of pineapple juice or milk.

Warm a nonstick skillet on medium-high heat. Measure about ⅓ cup of the batter onto the warm skillet. When bubbles start to appear on the top, after about 2 to 3 minutes, flip. Let the other side brown for about 2 minutes and remove from heat, and repeat.

Keep the cooked pancakes warm by placing them on a plate and covering them with a clean dishtowel or in an oven at 200°F until all the pancakes are cooked.

Once you've made all the pancakes, add the pineapple rings to the skillet and let brown for about 2 minutes, flip and cook for another two minutes.

Serve the browned pineapple over the pancakes and garnish with coconut. These pancakes are delicious topped with warm maple syrup or pineapple preserves.

Steel-Cut Oats

Chef Alex Bury offers this hearty dish. It's ideal to make it in advance for a warm, satisfying weekday breakfast. Make it on Sunday afternoon and you have morning meals for the week. This recipe makes a lot of oats, so you can either halve it or make the whole batch and freeze some for later.

SERVES 8
TIME: 50 minutes; 10 minutes active

2 cups uncooked whole-grain steel-cut oats
8 cups water
1 cinnamon stick, optional
2 medium apples, chopped
½ cup chopped nuts of your choice (almonds, pecans, and walnuts work well)
¼ cup raisins or other dried fruit
1½ cups of your favorite frozen berries
2 tablespoons ground cinnamon

Optional additions, added at the very end
1 cup puréed pumpkin with 1 teaspoon each nutmeg and clove
1 8-ounce can chopped pineapple in juice
1 chopped mango
½ cup peanut or almond butter

Put 8 cups of water in a very large pot, which will allow sufficient room to let the oats expand. Bring the water to a boil.

Pour the oats into the water, stirring.

Add the cinnamon stick.

Reduce the heat to low and stir every few minutes. If the oats are bubbling too much, turn the heat down. If they stick on the bottom, scrape and stir. Steel-cut oats are tough—they'll be fine no matter what you do to them!

After 20 minutes, add the chopped apple. Keep simmering and stirring for another 20 minutes. Turn off the heat. Stir in the nuts, raisins, ground cinnamon, and other optional ingredients. Stir often while cooling, remove the cinnamon stick, and then refrigerate.

Every morning, microwave a big bowl for your breakfast. Top with sliced bananas and more cinnamon if you like.

PRO-TIP: Keeps for 5 to 7 days in refrigerator. Pack in several small containers. You can freeze some of these small containers. That way you (and others in your family) can grab a container when you dash out the door and heat it in the office kitchen later. This helps you avoid the temptation of office donuts and cookies for breakfast.

Golden Country Biscuits and Gravy

I grew up in the South—and what that means is that biscuits and gravy are a standby for a hearty weekend breakfast. Biscuits and gravy were one of my grandmother's specialties (among many); this easy recipe will become one of your family's favorites too. You can make the biscuit dough in advance and freeze it, thawing it out later to make hot biscuits in a hurry.

MAKES 6
TIME: 30 minutes

Biscuits
1 cup whole wheat flour
1 cup all-purpose flour
½ teaspoon salt
1 tablespoon baking powder

4 tablespoons dairy-free margarine, like Earth Balance, plus an optional 1 tablespoon for brushing
1 cup plain, unsweetened soy or almond milk

Preheat oven to 400ºF. Set aside a nonstick baking sheet.

Combine all dry ingredients, then using a fork or pastry cutter cut in the margarine until crumbly and pieces are no larger than a pea. Add the soy or almond milk and stir until mixture is just thoroughly combined and all dry ingredients are mixed in, being careful not to overwork the dough.

Transfer the dough to a floured surface, and roll or pat it out to about ½-inch thick. Using a biscuit cutter or tumbler, cut out 6 biscuits and place on the nonstick baking sheet. You may need to reform the dough into a ball and press out again to make all the biscuits.

Optionally, brush the tops of the biscuits with a dab of margarine.

Bake for 15 minutes or until tops are golden brown. While the biscuits are in the oven, make the gravy.

To freeze: Shape the biscuits per instructions, place on a baking sheet, cover with plastic wrap, and put in the freezer. Once they've set long enough to hold their shape—about 4 hours to overnight—place into freezer bags or containers and store in the freezer until you're ready to eat them, up to a couple of months. When you're ready to eat them, remove from the freezer and place on baking sheets while the oven is preheating. Bake as per instructions, adding an extra 2 minutes if necessary to reach golden brown.

Gravy

2 tablespoons extra virgin olive oil

2 tablespoons all-purpose or whole wheat flour

2 tablespoons nutritional yeast

2 cups unsalted or low sodium vegetable broth or 2 cups water plus unsalted or low sodium bouillon paste sufficient to make 2 cups per package instructions

¼ teaspoon black pepper, more to taste

½ teaspoon dried powdered sage, optional

1 teaspoon salt, optional to taste

½ package meatless sausage crumbles, optional

Sprig of fresh sage for garnish

In a large skillet, toast the flour and nutritional yeast in olive oil on medium heat for 2 minutes or until it starts to brown, stirring regularly. Lower the heat and slowly add the broth, using a fork to crush any lumps that may form. Add the pepper, sage, salt, and crumbles, if using, and stir. Return the heat to medium until the gravy begins to bubble and thicken. Allow to simmer for 3 to 5 minutes, stirring regularly.

Place the biscuits on plates and spoon the gravy over them. Garnish with a sprig of fresh sage for a picture-perfect breakfast.

Savory Southern Sausage Biscuits

As a young girl, I loved heading out with my dad early on Saturday mornings to help him with various projects. We'd often stop at a fast-food joint for a sausage biscuit on the way. This recipe is a more healthful version that allows me to relive those memories without as much fat or as many calories. Wrap the warm sausage biscuits in napkins or foil and head out to greet your weekend with a full belly and a warm heart.

MAKES 6
TIME: 25 minutes

1 batch Golden Country Biscuits
   (page 134)
1 tablespoon dairy-free margarine,
   like Earth Balance, optional
1 package meatless sausage patties
   (Yves, LightLife, Amy's, Gardein),
   prepared according to package
   instructions

Dairy-free cheese, optional
   (I like Chao Cheese)

Prepare biscuits according to instructions in Golden Country Biscuits and Gravy recipe.

Brush the tops with margarine, if using. Allow the biscuits to cool to be able to handle. Cut the biscuits in half. Place a sausage patty on the bottom half of the biscuit. If using cheese, place the top of the biscuit on top of the cheese and heat in a toaster oven or warm oven for 2 to 3 minutes. If not, assemble sandwich style and enjoy.

Best Breakfast Pizzas, Mexican-style

Going MeatLess doesn't mean going fun-free. Yes, you can eat pizza for breakfast. Chef Alex Bury shows us how with these Mexican-style breakfast pizzas. Cumin and paprika season protein-rich tofu for a breakfast that will keep you fueled throughout the morning.

SERVES 4
TIME: 30 minutes; 15 active

1 large Yukon Gold potato, cubed
2 cups water
½ cup unsalted or low sodium vegetable broth or ½ cup water plus unsalted or low sodium bouillon paste sufficient to make ½ cup per package instructions
2 garlic cloves, finely chopped
½ onion, diced
2 cups chopped vegetables, like mushrooms, zucchini, broccoli, bell pepper, or other favorites

12 ounces silken tofu (I prefer Mori Nu, lowfat)
3 tablespoons scramble seasoning mix (page 138)
8 corn tortillas
1 15-ounce can refried beans (make sure they're meat-free)
1 package of Follow Your Heart or Daiya shredded vegan cheddar cheese, optional
1 15-ounce jar of your favorite salsa

Preheat oven to 400°F. Cover 2 cookie sheets with wax paper or aluminum foil and set aside.

Heat 2 cups of water in a large sauté pan or saucepot and bring to a boil.

Add the potato and cook for about 10 minutes until just tender. Remove from heat, strain, and discard the water.

Pour the vegetable broth or water into the pan or pot and heat on medium.

Add the potato, garlic, and onion and cook for 5 minutes. Add more water if needed to ensure the ingredients don't stick.

Add the vegetables and cook for 3 minutes.

Add the tofu and the seasoning mix. Stir everything very well and cook for 10 minutes, adding more water if necessary. Remove from heat.

Prepare the pizzas by spreading a layer of beans on each tortilla. Place the tortillas on the prepared cookie sheets. Top each tortilla with a layer of the tofu mixture, and top with grated cheese if using.

Bake for 10 minutes, until the topping is golden brown.

Top with salsa and enjoy!

Sunday Morning Scramble

There's nothing better in my house than a lazy Sunday morning break-fast. I love making Chef Alex's scramble with a side of potatoes and toast. You can make the spice mix in advance and keep a jar in the cupboard for easy access to make this a simple weekly staple.

SERVES 4
TIME: 20 minutes

Scramble Seasoning Mix
(*Make a big batch of this spice mix and keep in a jar in your cupboard for months*)

2⅔ cups nutritional yeast
2 tablespoons onion powder
2 tablespoons paprika
1 teaspoon celery seed
1 tablespoon cumin
1 tablespoon turmeric
3 tablespoons salt
1 teaspoon pepper

Scramble
12 ounces silken tofu (I like Mori-Nu)
16 ounces water-packed firm tofu, drained and pressed to remove water
4 tablespoons scramble seasoning mix
1 tablespoon extra virgin olive oil
1 cup of vegetables like broccoli, bell peppers, spinach, mushrooms, or carrots, chopped

In a medium bowl, mash the silken tofu and the firm tofu with a potato masher or your (freshly washed) hands.

Mix the scramble seasoning mix with the tofu mixture. Heat the oil in a large, nonstick pan over medium heat for 2 minutes. Add the tofu mixture and vegetables to the pan and sauté on medium heat for about 10 minutes. If the tofu starts sticking or getting dry, add a little water.

Taste before serving—some people prefer a stronger seasoning. If you fall into that camp, add an extra tablespoon of seasoning.

Serve with toast, home fries, and fresh fruit. Keep a bottle of hot sauce close by for those who like spicy food.

Handhelds

Delicious Deli Reuben

The sauce in this Reuben is so easy you won't believe it. You may want to make extra: as the name says, it's so delicious you'll want to put it on all of your sandwiches — you can use it to make a saucy, meatless Big Mac.

SERVES 4
TIME: 20 minutes active, 1.5 hours to allow time to marinate (or see pro-tip for a 10-minute version)

¼ cup dill pickle juice
⅛ cup soy sauce or tamari
1 8-ounce package tempeh
1 tablespoon extra virgin olive oil
½ onion, cut into half-moons
8 slices sandwich bread or 4 wraps

Sauce
¼ cup egg-free mayonnaise
  (I like Just Mayo)
2 tablespoons ketchup
2 tablespoons pickle relish

Topping
Dairy-free cheese, optional
Sauerkraut, to taste

Make the marinade: combine the pickle juice and soy sauce or tamari.

Slice the tempeh lengthwise into 8 to 10 strips and place into a shallow container. Pour the marinade over the tempeh and allow to soak for 30 minutes to 1 hour. The longer, the better.

Meanwhile, make the sauce: combine the mayonnaise, ketchup, and relish in a small bowl and stir until fully combined.

Preheat oven to 350°F.

Make the tempeh: After your tempeh has sufficiently marinated, add the oil to a medium-size frying pan. Sauté the onion in the oil until translucent, about 3 minutes. Add the tempeh and cook for ten minutes, flipping occasionally and adding a small amount of water or the juice from the marinade, if necessary, to ensure it doesn't stick.

Assemble the sandwiches: spread one-quarter of the spread on 4 slices of sandwich bread or wraps, add cheese, if using, sauerkraut, and then the tempeh. Line a cookie sheet with foil or wax paper, place on cookie sheet and toast in the oven for 10 minutes.

PRO-TIP: If you're short on time or just don't like cooking, skip the tempeh and the marinade (pickle juice, tamari, and onions) and pile a sandwich high with your favorite meatless deli slices such as Tofurky or Field Roast, then top with the sauce and sauerkraut. You can enjoy this delicious classic sandwich in a fraction of the time.

Chickpea of the Sea Salad Sandwiches

M ove over, tuna! The surprise ingredient in these sandwiches? Chick-peas. This versatile legume takes on the taste of the sea while deliv-ering a protein punch.

SERVES 2 TO 4
TIME: 10 minutes active, 1 hour to chill, optionally

1 15-ounce can chickpeas
¼ cup egg-free mayonnaise (I like Just
   Mayo)
2 tablespoons pickle relish
1 stalk celery, finely diced
2 green onions, finely chopped
Squeeze of fresh lemon juice
Salt and pepper
1 teaspoon nori flakes, optional

4 to 8 slices bread or 2 to 4 whole wheat
   wraps
Tomato slices, optional
4 large romaine lettuce leaves

Drain and rinse chickpeas. In a medium bowl, mash chickpeas with a po-tato masher or fork until crumbly. Combine remaining ingredients and mix well. Serve immediately by making sandwiches or wraps, or refrigerate for 1 hour or overnight. Makes 2 very stuffed or 4 lightly stuffed sandwiches or wraps.

> **PRO-TIP:** Mix in ¼ cup roasted, unsalted sunflower kernels to give the salad a little extra crunch and a blast of vitamins B and E.

Egg-Free Salad

This egg-free salad recipe is quick, easy, and delicious. Tofu soaks up the tangy mayonnaise, lemon juice, and the vinegary relish for a deli-style egg salad flavor. It's versatile, too. Use it as you would egg salad—as a sandwich filling or a salad topper.

SERVES 4
TIME: 10 minutes

16 ounces firm water-packed tofu, drained and rinsed

¼ cup egg-free mayonnaise (I like Just Mayo)

2 tablespoons pickle relish

2 tablespoons Dijon mustard

2 tablespoons lemon juice

½ teaspoon turmeric

1 tablespoon chopped fresh dill or 1 teaspoon dried dill

½ teaspoon paprika

¼ cup diced scallions

Salt and freshly ground pepper, to taste

Squeeze out excess water from tofu. With a potato masher or clean hands, mash the tofu in a bowl, leaving some texture. Add the remaining ingredients. Mix until combined. Chill for at least 30 minutes prior to serving.

PRO-TIP: Add additional seasonings to give it a twist, such as 1 teaspoon curry powder or 1 teaspoon cayenne pepper.

Chicken-Free Curry Salad Wraps

Here's another one from Chef Alex Bury's kitchen. Beyond Meat chicken-free strips have the same amount of protein as chicken but no cholesterol and no saturated fat. Serve a dollop of this curry salad on top of mixed greens or in a sandwich stuffed with other fresh vegetables for a lunch that's fast, super healthy, and super good for you! It's also a great party appetizer: serve on a large platter surrounded by crackers.

SERVES 4
TIME: 10 minutes

2 cups egg-free mayonnaise (I like Just
    Mayo)
4 tablespoons mild yellow curry powder
1 9-ounce package Beyond Meat
    Chicken-Free strips, either "Lightly
    Seasoned" or "Grilled," diced
2 stalks celery, washed and diced small,
    optional
½ yellow onion, finely diced, optional

½ cup golden raisins
1 teaspoon salt
½ teaspoon ground black pepper
1 teaspoon red chili flakes, optional
4 of your favorite wraps: lavash bread,
    flour tortillas, wraps, or large romaine
    lettuce leaves
Sliced, toasted almonds, chopped fresh
    cilantro, or lime wedges for garnish

Mix the mayonnaise and curry powder together in a large mixing bowl.

Add the remaining ingredients (except for the wraps). Mix well. Taste. Add more salt if desired, and/or red chili flakes if you like spicy food.

Place the bread, tortilla, wrap, or lettuce leaf on a clean surface. Add ½ cup curry salad. Roll up like a burrito.

PRO-TIP: Garnish with sliced, toasted almonds, chopped fresh cilantro, or lime wedges.

Rainbow Hummus Wraps

This is a great snack or lunch to make ahead of time, courtesy of Chef Alex Bury. You can make three or four wraps at a time and pack up the extras to take with you to the office or school. When you get the mid-day munchies, you'll have a healthy and satisfying snack waiting for you, so you can ignore the call of the vending machine!

SERVES 4
TIME: 10 minutes active

1 10-ounce tub of your favorite hummus (or one recipe of homemade hummus from the following recipe)

4 large flour tortillas or wraps (try whole wheat, spinach, or sundried tomato)

1 small salad bar to-go box from your favorite grocery store, filled with your

choice of cut vegetables: mushrooms, carrot and celery sticks, radish slices, spinach or romaine, sprouts, tomatoes, corn, shredded beets, zucchini, etc.

Optional: 1 package Tofurky or Field Roast Deli Slices

Spread a layer of hummus all over the tortilla. If using, add 2 to 3 deli slices. Sprinkle your vegetables over the spread toward the middle of the tortilla. Roll widthwise. Repeat. Use the whole package of hummus, all the vegetables and wraps, and store the extras to bring to work for a quick, healthy, and filling lunch.

PRO-TIP: Roll up, cut in half or using a serrated knife, cut into ½ inch slices as colorful hors d'oeuvres.

Homemade Hummus

Hummus makes an easy snack or sandwich filling and is widely available at most grocery and convenience stores. However, as Chef Alex Bury shows, it's incredibly easy to make and fun to customize to your liking: add fresh herbs for a flavor boost or peppers for more heat—the sky's the limit! Plus you can add as much or as little oil as you want if you're trying to cut calories.

MAKES 16 ounces
TIME: 10 minutes active

1 15-ounce can garbanzo beans
1 clove garlic, peeled
1 tablespoon white miso paste
Juice of ½ lemon, or about 2 tablespoons
¼ cup tahini
3 to 4 tablespoons extra virgin olive oil
Salt and fresh ground black pepper to taste

Optional add-ins
½ cup fresh dill, basil, or parsley leaves
¼ cup sun-dried tomatoes, rehydrated in water, drained, and chopped (oil-free variety)
¼ cup roasted red peppers, chopped (packed in water, not oil)
1 jalapeño, seeded and finely diced

Place all ingredients (except add-ins, if using) in a food processor with an "S" blade or high-powered blender, or place them in a high walled container and use an immersion blender.

Process until smooth. Add more oil or ⅛ to ¼ cup water if you want it thin (for dipping), or reduce liquid if you want it thick (for sandwich spreads). Gently stir in add-ins, if using.

Taste and add more lemon, miso, salt, or pepper if needed, and stir. Refrigerate for up to a week. Spread on bread or tortilla wraps; stir into fresh salad veggies; use as a dip for pretzels or vegetables

ute Tostadas

you're having one of those crazy weeks with too many work meetings and after-school events, you can count on this recipe to see you through. The basic dish from Chef Alex Bury uses only three ingredients. Try keeping them all in your pantry for "emergency" meal planning. It's filling, fresh, super healthy, and easy to "fancy up" if your in-laws are in town!

SERVES 4
TIME: 10 minutes active

1 jar of your favorite salsa
1 10-count package corn tortillas

1 15-ounce can refried beans (make sure they're meat-free)

If the tortillas are frozen, thaw them at room temperature or microwave for a few seconds until they're soft.

Open the can of beans and the jar of salsa.

Using a butter knife or small spatula, spread each tortilla with a layer of beans, using about 3 tablespoons per tortilla. The goal is to use the entire can of beans on the entire package of tortillas. Congratulations! You just did the hardest part.

Now you can microwave each tortilla for 30 seconds. If you're feeding everyone at once, place them on a cookie sheet or plate, stack them up like a layer cake and either bake in an oven that's 400°F for 20 minutes or microwave for 2 minutes.

Top warmed tortillas with a couple of spoonfuls of salsa. Roll up or fold in half, then repeat. No cholesterol and no oil means you can eat as many as you want!

Optional additions
- Toss some veggies on top when you microwave. Baby spinach is ideal because it cooks quickly, like the tortilla and beans. Chopped frozen vegetables or leftover cooked vegetables are perfect too!
- Layer all the bean tortillas in a casserole dish, sprinkle with vegetarian beef crumbles and dairy-free cheese (like Daiya or Follow Your Heart brands) and bake in the oven for 20 minutes.
- For a crispy tostada, first bake the tortilla(s) in an oven that's preheated to 350°F for 10 minutes, until they are crispy and lightly brown. Top with the refried beans and bake again. Finish with the salsa.

Soups

Souper Easy Split Pea Soup

This split pea soup is packed with goodness and is easy-peasy. Dry peas are a good source of iron, magnesium, phosphorus, potassium, and protein. According to the US Dry Pea & Lentil Council, they cost only about 7 cents per serving compared to chicken, which costs about 67 cents per serving. So dig in!

SERVES 4
TIME: 10 minutes active, 1½ hour cook time

6 cups water, low sodium vegetable broth, or 6 cups water plus low sodium bouillon paste sufficient to make 6 cups per package instructions

½ yellow or white onion, diced

2 cloves garlic, minced

2 cups dry split peas, rinsed and sorted for rocks

2 medium white potatoes, cubed

3 carrots, sliced

1 teaspoon liquid smoke, optional

1 teaspoon salt, or to taste

1 bay leaf

1 teaspoon dried thyme

½ teaspoon Herbes de Provence, optional

Croutons or grated carrots for garnish

In a large pot over medium high heat, add ¼ cup of stock or broth and onion. Steam fry the onion until translucent, about 3 minutes. Add the garlic and steam for another 2 minutes. Add remaining ingredients and bring mixture to a boil. Reduce to a simmer and stir periodically. The soup may foam, which is normal when cooking with split peas. Stir and lower heat slightly if this happens. Continue simmering until peas are tender, about an hour and a half.

Remove the bay leaf and serve. Or, if you prefer a smooth soup, transfer to a blender, or using an immersion blender, carefully pulse until

(Continues)

(*Continued*)

smooth. Return to the pot and heat until hot, adding more water if necessary.

Garnish with croutons or grated carrots for a splash of color.

PRO-TIP: Ladle soup into individual containers, allow to cool, seal containers, and freeze for up to three months for easy work lunches or quick homemade dinners!

New Mexican Chile Stew

Chile stew is one of my dad's specialties. The spicier, the better. How spicy is up to you. If you have roasted chiles, it's quick and easy, and paired with tortillas makes for a filling meal. The chiles create a deep, smoky flavor that'll make you want to sop up every drop with a warm tortilla.

SERVES 4
TIME: 40 minutes if using roasted peppers

2 tablespoons extra virgin olive oil or water

½ yellow onion, diced

3 to 4 cloves garlic, minced

1 15-ounce can diced tomatoes with juice or three large peeled, chopped red or green tomatoes with juice

1 tablespoon ground cumin

¼ cup Anaheim or Hatch peppers or 1 4-ounce can roasted green or Hatch chiles (more or less, according to your taste), roasted and peeled

2 white potatoes, cubed into 2-inch chunks

6 cups water, low sodium vegetable broth, or 6 cups water plus low sodium bouillon paste sufficient to make 6 cups per package instructions

1 package Boca crumbles, Beyond Beef Crumbles, Yves Ground Round, or texturized vegetable protein (TVP)

Salt to taste

1 tablespoon fresh cilantro, minced, for garnish, optional

Squeeze of lime juice, for garnish, optional

Sauté the onion in the oil or water on medium heat until translucent, about 3 minutes. Add the garlic and sauté one minute more. Add the tomatoes, cumin, peppers, potatoes, and water or broth and bring to a boil. Simmer for about 30 minutes, or until the potatoes are soft when pierced with a fork. Add the crumbles and simmer for 5 more minutes. Add salt to taste and garnish with cilantro and a squeeze of lime juice. Serve with warm tortillas.

PRO-TIP: Ladle soup into individual containers, allow to cool, seal containers, and freeze for up to three months for easy work lunches or quick homemade dinners!

PRO-TIP: You can use preroasted chiles in this recipe. If you want to roast your own, broil them for about 20 minutes at 400°F, then turn and broil for another 10 to 20 minutes or until the skin is blistered. Remove from oven and put in a sealable container, sealing the lid to trap the moisture and heat. Wearing gloves, remove one chile at a time from the bag, take out the seeds, and peel, after the chiles have cooled.

Creamy Cauliflower Soup

Cauliflower is not only packed with nutrients and becomes deliciously creamy when you cook it, it's also extremely versatile. And smart, apparently. Mark Twain called cauliflower a "cabbage with a college education." You will feel brilliantly satisfied after enjoying a bowl of this creamy, flavorful soup.

SERVES 4
TIME: 20 minutes

1 tablespoon extra virgin olive oil
½ yellow onion, diced
2 cloves garlic, minced
2 cups low sodium vegetable broth or 2 cups water plus low sodium bouillon paste sufficient to make 2 cups per package instructions
1 large head of cauliflower cut into florets, stems okay

½ teaspoon salt, optional
1 cup plain, unsweetened soy or almond milk
Pinch nutmeg
½ teaspoon black pepper
½ cup shredded dairy-free cheese, like Daiya, optional
Olive oil and roasted garlic, chopped, green onion tops, or chives for garnish

In a medium pot, sauté the onion in the oil on medium heat until translucent, about 3 minutes. Add garlic and sauté for 2 more minutes. Add broth and bring to a boil. Add cauliflower and salt, if using, and cook for about 10 minutes or until tender.

Add soy or almond milk, or use an immersion blender to purée until smooth and creamy, being careful not to splash yourself. A few chunks are okay if you prefer more texture. Transfer back to the pot and add the remaining ingredients. Cook for five minutes more or until hot, being careful not to let it boil.

Ladle into serving bowls and garnish with a drop of olive oil and roasted garlic, chopped green onion tops, or chives.

> **PRO-TIP:** Ladle soup into individual containers, allow to cool, seal containers, and freeze for up to three months for easy work lunches or quick homemade dinners!

Hearty Italian Minestrone

The cannellini beans give this traditional Italian soup fiber and protein. An easy weeknight dinner that makes great leftovers, this hearty soup is a great way to eat your vegetables on a cold winter night.

SERVES 4 to 6
TIME: 25 minutes

2 tablespoons extra virgin olive oil
½ medium yellow onion, diced
1 clove garlic, minced
1 15-ounce can diced tomatoes in juice
2 carrots, chopped
1 medium zucchini, chopped
5 cups water, low sodium vegetable broth
   or 5 cups water plus low sodium
   bouillon paste sufficient to make
   5 cups per package instructions
1 teaspoon salt
1 teaspoon ground pepper

1 cup alphabet, macaroni, or other pasta
½ bunch kale, torn into bite-size pieces
1 15-ounce can cannellini beans, rinsed,
   and drained
2 tablespoons tomato paste
1 teaspoon fresh thyme leaves or ½
   teaspoon dried
1 tablespoon chopped fresh basil or
   1 teaspoon dried
Chopped fresh basil or a sprig of parsley
   for garnish

In a large stockpot, sauté onion in olive oil on medium heat until translucent, about 3 minutes. Add garlic and continue to cook for another minute.

Add tomatoes, carrots, zucchini, water or broth, salt, and pepper. Bring to boil. Add pasta and cook for 7 to 9 minutes until al dente. Stir in kale, beans, tomato paste, thyme, and basil. Simmer for 5 minutes more.

Garnish with more chopped fresh basil or a sprig of parsley.

PRO-TIP: Ladle soup into individual containers, allow to cool, seal containers, and freeze for up to three months for easy work lunches or quick homemade dinners!

Luscious Lima Bean Soup

I f you hated lima beans when you were kid, get ready to fall in love. Lima beans are an inexpensive source of fiber and protein, and they're virtually fat-free. The liquid smoke adds an aroma that'll make you feel like you're sitting in front of a fireplace on a cold winter night all while enjoying a nourishing bowl of goodness.

SERVES 8
TIME: 2 hours and 5 minutes if using dried beans, 1 hour if using frozen.
Note: If using dried beans, allow at least 1 to 2 hours' soak time

1 pound dry lima beans plus 4 cups water
    or 1 pound frozen lima beans
¼ cup water for steam frying vegetables
4 large carrots, chopped
2 potatoes, cubed
½ cup medium yellow onion, diced
2 stalks celery, chopped
8 cups low sodium vegetable broth or
    8 cups water plus low sodium bouillon
    paste sufficient to make 8 cups per
    package instructions

2 tablespoons tomato paste
1 teaspoon dried oregano
1 teaspoon dried basil
½ teaspoon liquid smoke
Chopped fresh basil or oregano and a
    twist of fresh cracked black pepper for
    garnish

If using dried beans, bring 4 cups of water to a boil. Add dry lima beans, and boil for 2 to 3 minutes. Remove from heat, and allow the beans to soak, covered, for 1 to 2 hours to soften. Drain and rinse until water runs clear, discarding bean water.

In a soup pot, sauté vegetables in ¼ cup water until onions are translucent, about 3 minutes. Add lima beans, and sauté for another 2 to 3 minutes.

Add the remaining 8 cups water or broth and bring to a boil. Add tomato paste, oregano, basil, and liquid smoke if using, and allow soup to simmer on low for 1 to 1½ hours. Serve steaming hot.

Garnish with chopped fresh basil or oregano and a twist of fresh cracked black pepper.

PRO-TIP: Ladle soup into individual containers, allow to cool, seal containers, and freeze for up to three months for easy work lunches or quick homemade dinners!

Spiced Lentil Stew

Lentils, a great protein source, are super easy on the pocket book—but that's not the only reason to love this recipe from Chef Alex Bury: it's wholesome, nourishing, and easy. Chef Alex loves preparing this stew on a Sunday evening and putting some in the freezer to thaw and enjoy later in the week.

SERVES 4
TIME: 1 hour; 20 minutes active

2 medium yellow onions, diced
2 carrots, diced
¼ cup white wine or water
1 clove garlic, minced
2 stalks celery, diced
1 sweet potato or yam, peeled and diced
2 tablespoons ground cumin
1 cup dried brown lentils, rinsed
4 cups low sodium vegetable broth or
    4 cups water plus low sodium bouillon
    paste sufficient to make 4 cups per
    package instructions

1 28-ounce can plum tomatoes, chopped,
    with juice
½ head green cabbage, sliced thin
1 cinnamon stick or ¼ teaspoon ground
    cinnamon
½ bunch flat-leaf parsley, chopped
Salt to taste
Fresh ground black pepper to taste

Sauté the onions and carrots in wine or water in a large, heavy pot over medium-low heat for 8 minutes, stirring occasionally.

Add the garlic and celery and cook 2 minutes longer, stirring.

Add cumin and cook 1 minute longer.

Add the lentils, broth, tomatoes, cabbage, and cinnamon stick or ground cinnamon. Bring mixture to boil, reduce heat, and cook for 45 minutes, stirring occasionally.

Stir in the parsley and season to taste with salt and pepper. Remove the cinnamon stick before serving.

Ladle into bowls and garnish with chopped fresh parsley.

PRO-TIP: Ladle soup into individual containers, allow to cool, seal containers, and freeze for up to three months for easy work lunches or quick homemade dinners!

Mushroom Barley Soup

C hef Alex Bury gives this New York City deli classic a unique twist with wasabi powder. Fiber-rich barley adds a toothsome chewiness, earthy mushrooms provide a vitamin D boost, while dill adds fresh flavor and a hint of color. Enjoy with a crusty hunk of French bread for a filling meal.

SERVES 4
TIME: 1 hour; 10 minutes active

6½ cups water
½ cup barley
1 medium yellow onion, diced
2 tablespoons soy sauce or tamari
1 tablespoon dried parsley
2 teaspoons dried dill weed
1 teaspoon ground cumin
1 teaspoon garlic powder
½ teaspoon fresh cracked black pepper

¼ teaspoon wasabi powder, optional
1 pound fresh cremini or white button
    mushrooms, washed and sliced
1 medium cabbage, shredded, optional
    (you can use kale or any other leafy
    green vegetable instead, or omit
    altogether)
2 teaspoons chopped fresh dill for
    garnish, optional

Place the water, barley, onion, and seasonings in a large pot and stir. Cover and cook over medium heat for 30 minutes.

Add the mushrooms and cabbage and cook for another 30 minutes, stirring occasionally.

Ladle into soup bowls and garnish with fresh dill.

Butternut Squash Soup

When I think of fall foods, butternut squash comes to mind. Chef Alex Bury's delicious butternut squash soup is the perfect way to celebrate the fall bounty. Plus, it's chock full of vitamin C to help give you an immune boost as the weather changes.

SERVES 4
TIME: 40 minutes if using pre-roasted squash;
1 hour 20 minutes if using raw squash

2 medium yellow or white onions, diced

6 cloves garlic, peeled

1 tablespoon fresh ginger, peeled and minced

1 bay leaf

7 cups low sodium vegetable broth or 7 cups water plus low sodium bouillon paste sufficient to make 7 cups per package instructions

3 pounds butternut squash (or other winter squash), roasted and peeled (see Roasted Squash recipe, page 165)

or 3 pounds pre-cut winter squash, roasted on a greased baking sheet at 350°F for 40 minutes, turning once

½ cup orange juice

1 tablespoon orange zest

1 teaspoon ground cinnamon

1 tablespoon soy sauce or tamari

½ teaspoon nutmeg

Optional for garnish:
coconut milk, chives or green onions, roasted pumpkin seeds

In a large pot, combine the onions, garlic, ginger, bay leaf, and broth. Bring to a boil, then lower heat, and simmer gently for about 15 minutes.

Add the squash, orange juice, orange zest, cinnamon, soy sauce or tamari, and nutmeg. Simmer another 15 minutes.

Remove the bay leaf, transfer to a blender, or using an immersion blender, carefully pulse until smooth. Return to pot and reheat until hot. Season to taste.

Garnish with a swirl of coconut milk, chives or green onions, and roasted pumpkin seeds.

Variations: You can substitute half of the squash with sweet potatoes, yams, or carrots or a mixture of them. You can also use 2 tablespoons curry powder instead of the cinnamon and nutmeg.

PRO-TIP: Ladle soup into individual containers, allow to cool, seal containers, and freeze for up to three months for easy work lunches or quick homemade dinners!

Vegetable Bisque

B isque usually connotes a creamy, rich seafood soup. Chef Alex Bury's vegetable bisque recipe has all the creamy goodness of a bisque without all the fat. On top of that, it's perfect for slow cookers and will warm up your home on cold winter days.

SERVES 4
TIME: 1 hour, 10 minutes

7 cups low sodium vegetable broth or 7 cups water plus low sodium bouillon paste sufficient to make 7 cups per package instructions

3 large shallots or 1 large yellow onion, diced

1 leek, white and light green parts only, washed very well and chopped

2 medium Yukon gold potatoes, scrubbed and cubed

1 large celery root, peeled and chopped

½ medium head of cauliflower, chopped

Kernels from 1 large or 2 small ears of fresh corn or 1 cup frozen or canned corn

2 large cloves garlic, minced

3 sprigs fresh thyme or 1 teaspoon dried thyme leaves

2 bay leaves

Salt and fresh cracked black pepper to taste

2 tablespoons minced fresh chives for garnish, optional

Start the broth heating in a very large soup pot or your slow cooker.

Prep and chop the vegetables.

Throw everything into the pot except for the salt, pepper, and fresh chives.

If using the stovetop: bring to a boil, then simmer for at least an hour until everything is falling-apart tender.

If using a slow cooker: cook on high for 4 hours, or low for 8, until everything is very tender.

Remove the bay leaves, transfer to a blender, or using an immersion blender, carefully pulse until smooth. Return to pot and reheat until hot. If you want it thicker, add an arrowroot or cornstarch slurry (see Pro-Tip).

Add salt and pepper to taste. Spoon into bowls (dark colored if you have them) and top with the chives.

PRO-TIP: Want to know how to make a thickening slurry? Hint: this works only for foods that will be heated. Mix 2 tablespoons arrowroot or cornstarch with ¼ cup *cold* water in a small bowl. Gently stir this mixture into your sauce or soup. Bring to a simmer. The starches will not thicken until they reach a simmer. If it's still not thick enough, repeat, but always give it a few minutes before adding more to allow the slurry to reach its full thickening potential!

Lentil Soup

Okay, so you know lentils are a great source of protein, but did you know they're a good source of calcium too? This lentil soup is brothy, yet the potatoes and vegetables add substance and heartiness. It's quick and easy enough for a weeknight meal, and it's especially filling when paired with maple corn muffins (adjoining page).

SERVES 2 to 4 (2 large bowls, 4 cups)
TIME: 35 minutes

¼ cup water
½ yellow or white onion, diced
2 cloves garlic, minced
3 carrots, chopped
2 medium potatoes, diced
1 15-ounce can of diced tomatoes with juice
4 cups low sodium vegetable broth or 4 cups water plus low sodium bouillon paste sufficient to make 4 cups per package instructions

1 cup frozen mixed vegetables
1 tablespoon fresh oregano (or 1 teaspoon dried), chopped
1 teaspoon fresh thyme (or ½ teaspoon dried), chopped
1 cup brown or green lentils, dried
Salt or pepper to taste
Wilted spinach leaves for garnish

Warm the water in a large pot over medium heat and add the onion to steam until soft and turning translucent, about 3 minutes.

Add the garlic, carrots, and potatoes. Cook for one minute, stirring, so the garlic doesn't brown.

Add the remaining ingredients.

Raise heat and bring the mixture to a boil, then partially cover the pot and reduce heat to a simmer. Cook for 25 to 30 minutes, or until the lentils are tender.

Add salt and pepper to taste.

Serve garnished with wilted spinach leaves.

PRO-TIP: Ladle soup into individual containers, allow to cool, seal containers, and freeze for up to three months for easy work lunches or quick homemade dinners!

Sides and Sauces

Maple Corn Muffins

Corn muffins are a quick bread that make a great accompaniment to so many meals: soups, salads, and more. Chef Alex Bury's are perfectly crumbly with a hint of sweetness from the maple syrup. Make an extra batch to store in the freezer.

MAKES 12
TIME: 30 minutes

1 cup whole wheat flour
1 cup corn flour or fine cornmeal
Pinch salt, optional
1 tablespoon baking powder
½ cup maple syrup
1 cup plain, unsweetened soy or almond milk
2 tablespoons Ener-G Egg Replacer mixed with 2 tablespoons water or

1 flax egg (1 tablespoon flax meal mixed with 2 tablespoons water) stirred vigorously
Optional: 3 tablespoons dried cranberries, chopped pecans, and/or corn kernels for garnishes

Preheat oven to 375°F. If using regular muffin tins, lightly grease and set aside.

Mix all dry ingredients in a bowl and make a well in the center.

Pour wet ingredients into well and mix thoroughly, then stir in garnishes (if using). The mixture will be very runny.

Pour into silicone muffin pans or lightly greased regular pans and bake for 15 to 20 minutes, or until tops are golden brown.

Fresh Spring Rolls with Peanut Sauce

Fresh spring rolls look so elegant and Chef Alex Bury has found that when teaching cooking classes everyone is surprised by how easy they are to make. Her fresh spring rolls make a delicious appetizer or finger food for parties. If you've never worked with rice paper wrappers, you may need to practice with a couple before you get it right. The trick is to dampen the paper but not to let it soften too much or else it may fall apart. Don't worry—you've got this!

MAKES 8
TIME: 25 minutes

Filling
1 head green cabbage, shredded
   (try Napa cabbage if you can find it)
2 carrots, grated
2-inch piece of ginger, peeled and finely
   chopped
2 cloves of fresh garlic, finely chopped
⅓ bunch cilantro, chopped, optional
4 to 5 mint leaves, chopped, optional

¼ cup lime juice
2 tablespoons soy sauce or tamari
1 teaspoon dried, ground coriander
1 8-ounce package marinated tempeh cut
   lengthwise into 8 strips (I like Tofurky
   Coconut Curry)
8 round rice paper wrappers (found in
   Asian markets)

In a medium bowl, mix the cabbage and carrots together.

In a small bowl whisk the ginger, garlic, herbs, lime juice, soy sauce or tamari, and coriander together.

Pour the sauce over the carrots and cabbage, and toss to coat. Taste and adjust seasonings to your liking. You can use it right away, but if you have time to allow it to marinate for an hour, the flavor intensifies.

When you're ready to assemble the rolls, dip each rice paper wrapper in warm water until it begins to soften for about 15 to 20 seconds, one at a time.

Once you've softened the wrapper, place it on a clean, dry towel.

Put one tempeh strip and ⅓ cup of filling at the bottom of the roll, leaving at least an inch on both sides.

Roll from the bottom, and when you've rolled it once completely, fold the sides in, and continue rolling until it's completely rolled. The rice paper should stick to itself to seal.

Serve on a bed of shredded cabbage with peanut sauce (adjoining page) and a sprig of mint or cilantro.

(*Continues*)

(*Continued*)

Peanut Dipping Sauce

This delicious peanut sauce from Chef Alex Bury can be used as a dip for spring rolls or tossed with shredded cabbage and carrots for an Asian-inspired slaw. Crumbling some crushed peanuts over the top adds some crunch and texture.

MAKES 1½ cups
TIME: 15 minutes

2 cloves garlic
1-inch piece of fresh ginger, peeled
⅓ cup fresh cilantro, mint, or Italian parsley leaves (or some combination of the three)
1 tablespoon maple syrup or agave nectar
2 tablespoons soy sauce or tamari
2 tablespoons rice vinegar or apple cider vinegar

½ teaspoon chili powder, optional
1 tablespoon toasted sesame oil
½ cup natural peanut butter, smooth or chunky
1 cup warm water
½ cup chopped scallions

Purée the garlic, ginger, and herbs in a food processor until they're finely chopped.

Add everything else except water and scallions.

With the processor running, pour in the water.

Taste and adjust seasoning if necessary. Remove from the food processor and stir in the scallions.

Maple Glazed Brussels Sprouts

This is a great basic recipe for Brussels sprouts and any winter root vegetable such as carrots and turnips. Chef Alex Bury shares that the sesame oil, ginger, maple syrup, and soy sauce are the important seasonings that can be used for any sautéed vegetable. Roasted vegetables are wonderful served with holiday meals and a great way to get kids to try—and like—Brussels sprouts.

SERVES 4
TIME: 25 minutes

½ yellow onion, sliced

1 carrot, cut in matchsticks or coins

2 cups Brussels sprouts, washed, ends removed, cut in half lengthwise

1 tablespoon fresh ginger, peeled and chopped

1½ tablespoons soy sauce or tamari

1 tablespoon maple syrup

1 tablespoon toasted sesame oil

Heat ½ cup of water in a large sauté pan. Add the onion, carrots, and Brussels sprouts.

Steam-sauté for about 10 minutes. Stay close to the pan. Allow the water to evaporate at least once, so the cut surfaces of the vegetables can caramelize on the dry pan. That brings out their natural sugars. They need only a minute or so on the dry heat, and then you'll need to add more water. This cooking method works for all vegetables and is a delicious alternative to cooking in oil.

Add the ginger and cook for another couple of minutes.

When the Brussels sprouts are almost done—still firm but no longer crunchy—add the soy sauce or tamari, maple syrup, and sesame oil. Stir well, bring to a boil, and then turn off the heat.

Herb-Roasted Winter Vegetables

Winter vegetables that may be bland or earthy often taste sweet when roasted. These foods are high in natural sugars and roasting brings out their natural sweetness. Chef Alex Bury adds fresh rosemary and thyme to create a fragrant aroma that makes them irresistible. These are a perfect holiday side dish or flavor addition to any fall or winter entrée.

SERVES 6
TIME: 40 minutes

2 cups bite-size cauliflower florets, each halved lengthwise

2 cups Brussels sprouts, washed, ends removed, cut in half lengthwise

2 medium carrots, cut into sticks

1 medium yam or sweet potato, diced

2 tablespoons extra virgin olive oil

1 tablespoon chopped fresh rosemary

2 teaspoons chopped fresh thyme

Salt and pepper to taste

1 tablespoon balsamic vinegar

2 tablespoons chopped fresh parsley

Preheat oven to 450°F.

Place cauliflower, Brussels sprouts, carrots, and yam or sweet potato in a roasting dish, preferably glass or ceramic.

Add the oil, rosemary, and thyme, and toss to coat. Season with salt and pepper.

Roast for 30 minutes, turning 2 or 3 times with a spatula to prevent sticking. The vegetables are done when they're tender and dark brown.

Toss with balsamic vinegar, sprinkle with parsley, and add more fresh chopped herbs if desired.

Roasted Root Vegetable Salad

T he winter season is long, and root vegetables are aplenty. When I've run out of ideas for how to use them, I'll roast and toss them into a salad. It's colorful, hearty, and a nice way to bring a little spring into your winter. The dressing is an easy staple you can keep on hand for any greens or vegetables.

SERVES 2
TIME: 40 minutes

Your choice of 2 cups of winter root
  vegetables (carrots, Tokyo turnips,
  beets, turnips), chopped into cubes
1 tablespoon extra virgin olive oil
Salt to taste
½ teaspoon fresh or ⅛ teaspoon dried
  thyme
½ teaspoon fresh or ⅛ teaspoon dried
  rosemary
Head of lettuce washed and torn or 4 cups
  of your choice of salad greens
¼ cup chopped walnuts

Dressing
¼ cup extra virgin olive oil
3 tablespoons balsamic vinegar
3 tablespoons red wine or water
¼ teaspoon mustard seeds
¼ teaspoon black pepper
¼ teaspoon salt

Preheat oven to 450°F.

Place vegetables in a roasting dish. Drizzle with olive oil, add the salt and herbs, and toss.

Roast for 30 minutes, turning two or three times with a spatula to prevent sticking. The vegetables are done when they're tender and dark brown.

Meanwhile, wash the lettuce or salad greens and prepare the dressing. Blend the oil, vinegar, wine, or water well. Then whisk in the mustard seeds, pepper, and salt.

Once the vegetables have finished cooking, allow to cool, and then toss with the lettuce, walnuts, and dressing, and serve.

Roasted Squash

I've seen Chef Alex Bury demo this recipe—if we can call it that—at least half a dozen times. Of course, all her food is amazing, but every time she showcases this trick, a collective "ahh" falls over the room. This is the simplest recipe imaginable. No poking, peeling, slicing, or chopping involved.

SERVES 4, using 1 large squash
TIME: 40 minutes

1 to 2 of your favorite seasonal hard
   squashes like butternut, kabocha,
   or acorn

Preheat oven to 400°F.

Take the sticker off the squash. Rinse the squash and place it on a piece of foil on a baking dish or cookie sheet. Bake for 20 minutes, turn over, and bake for another 20 minutes. Test with a knife. When the knife slips in easily, it's done.

Allow to cool (I often slice it in half at this point so it cools faster, being careful to avoid the steam). Scoop out the seeds. The skin will peel away easily.

Serving suggestions: sprinkle squash slices with soy sauce or tamari and eat with rice, mash with a fork and top with a tablespoon of maple syrup and a sprinkle of cinnamon, or turn it into soup (see page 155).

Quinoa and Navy Bean Salad

C hef Alex combines protein-rich quinoa and navy beans to create a re-
freshing, yet filling salad. Don't like navy beans? Don't worry: you can
use any kind of bean you like. The lime juice adds tang to the subtle heat of
the chiles while the cilantro and cumin provide Latin flavors. Enjoy it warm
or cold—the choice is yours!

SERVES 4 to 6
TIME: 35 minutes

1 cup water
⅓ cup dry quinoa
1 tablespoon fresh lime juice
1 teaspoon ground cumin
1 teaspoon ground coriander
1 tablespoon finely chopped fresh cilantro
2 tablespoons minced green onions
2 cups cooked navy beans or 1 15-ounce
    can, drained

2 cups diced tomatoes or 1 15-ounce can,
    drained
1 cup diced red bell pepper
2 teaspoons minced fresh (or canned)
    green chiles
Salt and black pepper to taste
Chopped fresh cilantro for garnish

Bring the water to a boil in a saucepan. Add quinoa, cover, and simmer
about 10 to 15 minutes until all the water is absorbed. Fluff with a fork.
Cool 15 minutes.

Meanwhile, in a large bowl, combine the lime juice, cumin, coriander,
cilantro, and green onions. Stir in the beans, tomatoes, bell peppers, and
chiles.

Add the cooled quinoa, mix well, and season with salt and pepper to
taste.

Garnish with chopped, fresh cilantro.

Curried Red Lentil and Cauliflower Salad

Full of both fiber and protein, this salad from Chef Alex Bury makes a hearty lunch or dinner (serve it as a side with baked tofu [page 173] or braised tempeh [page 175]). It's quick, too: red lentils cook up fast and add color to this festive salad. The balsamic vinegar, apple, and currants provide a hint of sweetness.

SERVES 4
TIME: 25 minutes

2 cups water or low sodium vegetable broth or 2 cups water plus low sodium bouillon paste sufficient to make 2 cups per package instructions
2 cups red lentils, rinsed
1 medium onion, diced
2 cloves garlic, minced
¼ cup white wine or water

1 to 2 tablespoons curry powder, to taste
1 medium head of cauliflower cut into florets
1 small apple, cored and chopped
¼ cup currants
1 tablespoon balsamic vinegar
1 tablespoon soy sauce or tamari

In a medium stockpot, bring the water or stock to a boil. Add the lentils and lower to a simmer. Cook until lentils are tender and still whole, about 10 to 15 minutes.

Meanwhile, in a medium pan, sauté the onions and garlic in the wine or water for 3 minutes. Add the curry powder and the cauliflower florets. Cook, stirring, until the cauliflower is tender, yet still crisp.

When the lentils are done, in a medium bowl combine them with the spiced cauliflower, apple, and currants. Season with the balsamic vinegar and soy sauce or tamari.

Two-Grain Pilaf with Wild Mushrooms

W hole grains, whole grains—everyone's telling us to eat more whole grains. Good news: this recipe is a delicious way to mix up the grains in your diet. Chef Alex Bury pairs nutty wild rice with chewy barley and earthy mushrooms to please your palate, scrub your arteries, and give you a vitamin D boost. All those benefits aside, you'll love the savory flavor. Serve as a side to baked tofu [page 173] and sautéed greens, and you'll be full of so much nutrient goodness you won't know what to do with all your energy.

SERVES 4
TIME: 1 hour; 15 minutes active

½ cup hulled barley
½ cup dry wild rice
¾ cup water
1⅔ cups low sodium vegetable broth or
    1⅔ cups water plus low sodium
    bouillon paste sufficient to make
    1⅔ cups per package instructions
1 tablespoon dried thyme
1 teaspoon dried marjoram

1 teaspoon black pepper
¼ teaspoon salt
1 medium carrot, thinly sliced into coins
2 to 3 tablespoons white wine or water
1 cup sliced or chopped fresh button or
    cremini mushrooms
1 stalk celery, diced
1 medium white or yellow onion, diced
Sprig of thyme for garnish

In a large saucepan combine barley, wild rice, water, vegetable broth, thyme, marjoram, pepper, and salt. Cook over high heat until mixture comes to a full boil. Reduce heat to low and simmer.

Cover and continue cooking until the water is absorbed and the barley and rice are tender, about 40 to 45 minutes.

Meanwhile, sauté the carrot in wine or water for 2 minutes. Add the mushrooms, celery, and onion. Continue cooking, stirring occasionally, until the celery is tender, yet crisp.

Once the rice and barley have fully absorbed the liquid, stir in the vegetable mixture. Serve hot, garnished with a sprig of thyme.

Mediterranean Chickpeas

This recipe from Chef Alex Bury makes an excellent side or an entrée when served over couscous or rice. While the versatile chickpea has a starring role, tomatoes, olives, artichokes, and oregano combine to provide a bold, rich flavor.

SERVES 4
TIME: 40 minutes

1 medium yellow onion, diced
3 cloves garlic, minced
2 tablespoons extra virgin olive oil
3 cups cooked chickpeas,
    or 1½ 15-ounce cans
1 10-ounce package frozen chopped
    spinach, defrosted, or 1 large bunch
    fresh spinach, washed, and chopped
1 28-ounce can crushed tomatoes in juice
1 cup chopped fresh tomatoes
1 teaspoon crushed red pepper flakes

1 teaspoon dried oregano
Juice of 1 lemon or 2 tablespoons
1 6½-ounce jar artichoke hearts, rinsed
    and roughly chopped
¼ cup sundried tomatoes, either soaked
    in warm water until soft or packed in
    oil
Salt and black pepper to taste
¼ cup chopped, pitted Kalamata olives,
    optional
2 tablespoons capers, optional

Sauté the onion and garlic in the oil in a large saucepan over medium heat until the onion is tender.

Add the chickpeas, spinach, tomatoes, pepper flakes, and oregano. Cover and simmer for 30 minutes. Add the lemon juice, artichokes, sundried tomatoes, salt, and pepper.

Add olives and capers if using.

Delicious served right away when it's still warm, but it also makes a nice cold salad for lunch.

Tomato and Black Bean Salsa

C hef Alex Bury's fresh salsa can really be made of anything—use your imagination and what you have on hand—change up the beans and use kidney or pinto, shred some cabbage or add some corn. Serve as a condiment to Mexican or Southwestern dishes, as a filling for sandwiches or wraps, or as a dip for tortilla chips.

SERVES 4 to 6
TIME: 15 minutes

1½ cups ripe fresh tomatoes, diced
1 cup red pepper, seeds removed and
    diced
½ cup red onion, diced
⅓ cup green onions, thinly sliced
¼ cup jalapeño pepper, seeds removed
    and diced, optional
¼ cup freshly chopped cilantro, optional
1 tablespoon garlic, minced

¾ cup cooked black beans (about ½ of a
    15-ounce can)
1 to 2 tablespoons lime juice, to taste
Salt and freshly ground black pepper, to
    taste

In a medium bowl, combine the tomatoes, red pepper, red onion, green onions, jalapeño pepper, cilantro, and garlic, and toss well to combine.

Add the black beans and gently mix in.

Season to taste with lime juice, salt, and pepper and toss lightly.

PRO-TIP: You can add in corn kernels, diced mango, pineapple, or tomatillos for new flavors.

Creamy Cashew Gravy

C ashews are the surprise ingredient in this easy, creamy gravy. Not only
    do cashews add protein, but they're also good for your heart. Cashews
are soft enough that when ground up with liquid, they provide a rich, vel-
vety base. Combined with miso and mushrooms for an umami flavor ("the
fifth taste," which was coined in Japan to describe a pleasant, savory taste
sensation), the gravy is perfect with mashed potatoes, over a holiday roast,
or even as the filling in a pot pie.

MAKES 4 cups
TIME. 15 minutes

⅔ cup raw, unsalted cashews, soaked in
    water for an hour to overnight if time
    allows
¼ cup nutritional yeast
⅓ cup arrowroot powder or cornstarch
1 tablespoon red miso
2 tablespoons soy sauce or tamari
3½ cups water, red wine, low sodium
    vegetable broth, or 3½ cups water plus
    low sodium bouillon paste sufficient to
    make 3½ cups per package
    instructions

1 cup sliced sautéed mushrooms, optional
½ cup diced sautéed onions, optional
½ teaspoon rubbed sage, optional
Salt and black pepper to taste

Add all ingredients to a high-powered blender or food processor and purée
until creamy and smooth. If you're using a conventional blender, you may
need to take a few extra minutes to blend the nuts.

Taste and adjust the seasonings.

If the mixture is too thick, add a little water; if it's too thin, combine 1
tablespoon arrowroot or cornstarch with 2 tablespoons cold water, mix
vigorously, and add to the cashew mixture. Add to a large saucepan.
Warm until the mixture just begins to bubble, stirring frequently. Remove from heat.

PRO-TIP: For a mushroom-cashew gravy, sauté 1 cup sliced
mushrooms and onions in wine or water, and then add the gravy to
the pot. Cook until thick and the mixture just begins to bubble,
stirring frequently. Remove from heat.

Tempting Tennessee BBQ Sauce

C hef Alex Bury's homemade barbecue sauce makes a real treat for cookouts or summer celebrations. It's an ideal marinade or sauce on tofu, seitan, and veggie burgers.

MAKES 2 cups
TIME: 10 minutes

½ cup tomato paste
½ cup apple cider vinegar
¼ cup maple syrup
¼ cup Jack Daniels, bourbon, or water
¼ cup soy sauce or tamari

2 cloves garlic
1 inch knob of ginger, peeled
1 tablespoon dry mustard
¼ teaspoon ground black pepper
¼ teaspoon cayenne pepper

Combine all ingredients in a food processor or blender and purée until smooth. Place in a sealed jar and keep refrigerated for up to 2 weeks.

Entrées

Baked Tofu

Tofu can have a bad rap (see my story on page 3). This recipe will flip that notion on its head. Once you see how easy and delicious Chef Alex Bury's baked tofu is, you'll never buy the packaged stuff from the store again. It's perfect in stir-fries and salads, barbecued, with noodles and a peanut sauce, and more—use your imagination!

SERVES 4
TIME: 30 to 40 minutes; most inactive

1 pound, firm or extra-firm water-packed tofu
Cooking spray oil
2 tablespoons white wine, optional
1 tablespoon extra virgin olive oil
2 tablespoons soy sauce or tamari
2 tablespoons nutritional yeast

Optional
1 tablespoon curry powder or
  1 tablespoon dried Italian herbs, added when tossing with the oil
2 tablespoons sriracha or other hot sauce when the tofu comes out of the oven

Preheat oven to 350°F.

Rinse the tofu, press water out (see Pro-tip), then cut into ½-inch cubes. The smaller the cubes, the faster it will bake.

Lightly spray a cookie sheet with spray oil.

In a bowl, toss the tofu cubes with the wine, if using, and oil. Place on prepared cookie sheet.

Bake at 350°F for about 20 minutes, flip, and bake for 10 minutes more until cubes become golden brown.

Remove from the oven and immediately toss with the tamari and nutritional yeast and other seasonings, if using.

The tofu is delicious warm like this, or it can be chilled overnight, which makes it even firmer.

(Continues)

(*Continues*)

PRO-TIP: To press water out of tofu, drain it and gently squeeze it between your palms. Then place the tofu on a plate on top of several paper towels. Place more paper towels on top of the tofu. Place another plate or cutting board on top of the tofu and weigh it down with a pot, books, or cans of beans for 10 to 15 minutes or up to 1 hour. The longer you press it, the more excess water you'll be able to drain and the more toothsome the texture will be.

Braised Tempeh

B raising protein and fiber-rich tempeh allows it to soak up the marinade, making it rich and flavorful. This tempeh from Chef Alex Bury can be served as the main course in a meal surrounded by vegetables, or in a salad or stir-fry. Try it on pizzas, crumbled in county gravy (page 134), or on top of rice with a side of greens. It's very versatile.

SERVES 2 to 4
TIME: 40 minutes

1 8-ounce package tempeh, any type, cut into 1-inch cubes

1 tablespoon extra virgin olive oil

1 cup water

1 cup wine (white or red), beer, water, or low sodium vegetable broth; divided into two equal portions of ½ cup each

1 tablespoon soy sauce or tamari

1 tablespoon maple syrup

2 cloves garlic, sliced lengthwise

1 tablespoon Italian seasoning

In a medium pan over medium to high heat, sauté the tempeh in the oil.

When it gets golden brown, add half the wine, beer, broth, or water. Simmer for another few minutes until the liquid has cooked down.

Pour all the other ingredients into the pan over the tempeh. Bring to a boil, and then turn down to a simmer. Gently cook until most of the liquid has been absorbed and the tempeh cubes are tender, about 20 minutes.

Vitality Bowl

This is inspired by the Dragon Bowl, a menu staple at New York City's Angelica Kitchen. It's hearty, delicious, and colorful—a clean meal that makes you feel healthier just looking at it. Choose whatever vegetables and beans you have on hand or that are in season.

SERVES 2
TIME: 35 MINUTES

1 bunch greens (kale, collards, or chard), cut into bite-size pieces

2 cups cooked seasonal vegetables like broccoli, squash, and cauliflower

1 15-ounce can beans of your choice or 2 cups cooked beans (chickpeas, black-eyed peas, black beans, pinto beans, and red beans all make good choices)

2 cups cooked brown rice (or grain of your choice)

Miso Tahini Dressing
2 heaping tablespoons tahini
1 tablespoon miso
¾ cup warm water
1 teaspoon dried dill

Steam greens and seasonal vegetables until tender, about 5 minutes.

To make the sauce, combine tahini and miso then slowly add warm water. The sauce will thicken at first. Smooth out lumps, and then add remaining water and dill.

Fill two bowls with half of the rice, greens, beans, and seasonal vegetables, and then pour the dressing over to taste.

Garnish with a sprinkle of dill or sesame seeds.

Easy Spring Risotto

There's nothing better than a spring risotto, and the more I make this recipe, the easier it gets. It requires a lot of stirring, but don't let that intimidate you. You can substitute your favorite vegetables, such as fresh peas in spring or butternut squash in the fall, in place of the mushrooms and asparagus for a great meal any time of the year. Don't let risotto's notorious difficulty scare you—it's all about stirring regularly!

SERVES 2
TIME: 40 minutes

1 tablespoon extra virgin olive oil
½ cup finely chopped yellow or white onion
1 clove garlic, minced
½ cup Arborio rice
1½ cups water, 1½ cups low sodium vegetable broth, or 1½ cups water plus low sodium bouillon paste sufficient to make 1½ cups per package instructions

Half bunch—six or so stalks—asparagus, ends trimmed off and cut into 1-inch lengths
1 cup chopped white button or cremini mushrooms
1 teaspoon dried thyme
1 teaspoon dried oregano
1 teaspoon fresh lemon juice
Salt and pepper to taste
Spring of thyme for garnish

In a large saucepan, heat the olive oil on medium. Add the onions and cook for 3 minutes until translucent. Add the garlic and cook for 2 more minutes. Reduce heat to low.

Add the rice, and then slowly begin adding water or broth ½ cup at a time, stirring regularly. Once the water is absorbed, add more. Once you've added 1 cup of the water, add the asparagus, mushrooms, thyme, oregano, lemon juice, and salt and pepper to taste. Add the rest of the water and continue stirring regularly. Serve once all the water has been absorbed and the risotto is soft and creamy, about 30 minutes. Garnish with a sprig of thyme.

Herbed Italian Stuffed Shells

I f you're new to tofu or introducing someone else to it, this is the gateway recipe. You and your dinner guests won't believe the ricotta in this recipe is actually a blend of tofu and herbs. Make an extra serving: you're going to want leftovers. Some folks may argue that it's even better the next day!

SERVES 4
TIME: 45 minutes

½ box of jumbo pasta shells

1 10-ounce package frozen chopped spinach, thawed and drained or 1 bunch fresh spinach, washed

1 pound firm water-packed tofu, drained and squeezed

1 tablespoon sugar or agave nectar

¼ cup plain, unsweetened soy or almond milk

½ teaspoon garlic powder

2 tablespoons lemon juice

3 teaspoons minced fresh basil

2 teaspoons salt

1 25-ounce jar of your favorite tomato sauce or use Quick and Easy Pasta Marinara (page 181)

½ cup dairy-free cheese, optional

Chopped fresh basil or organo for garnish

Cook the noodles according to the package directions. Drain and set aside to cool.

Preheat oven to 400°F.

Squeeze the spinach as dry as possible and set aside. If using fresh spinach, blanch in boiling water for about a minute, strain well, and set aside.

Place the tofu, sugar or agave, milk, garlic powder, lemon juice, basil, and salt in a food processor or blender and blend until smooth. Stir in (don't blend) the spinach.

Cover the bottom of a 13 x 9-inch baking dish with a thin layer of tomato sauce. Spoon 2 to 3 tablespoons of the tofu filling into each shell and place in the baking dish. Top the stuffed shells with the remaining tomato sauce and dairy-free cheese, if using. Bake for 20 to 25 minutes.

Garnish with chopped, fresh basil or oregano.

Polenta Lasagna

This recipe by Chef Alex Bury is a great source of complex carbohydrates, protein from the chickpeas, vitamins and fiber from the vegetables, and antioxidants from the tomatoes. All that for pennies from your bank account and just a few minutes out of your busy day. Serve it with a big salad and eat the entire pan!

SERVES 4
TIME: 30 minutes

1 tablespoon extra virgin olive oil
1 tube cooked polenta
1 25-ounce jar of your favorite meat- and dairy-free tomato sauce or use Quick and Easy Pasta Marinara (page 181)
1 15-ounce can garbanzo beans, drained and rinsed
1 medium zucchini, sliced thin, or 15-ounce bag of baby spinach, washed

Optional additions
½ cup meat-free beef crumbles or chicken strips, sautéed lightly in olive oil
½ cup sliced mushrooms
½ of a 15-ounce can of water-packed artichoke hearts, drained
3 tablespoons nutritional yeast
¼ cup shredded dairy-free cheese
1 tablespoon Italian seasoning
1 tablespoon crushed red pepper flakes

Preheat oven to 400°F. Lightly coat a casserole dish with oil.

Slice the polenta into thin slices.

Layer the polenta with the sauce, beans, and vegetables. If using crumbles, chicken strips, mushrooms, or artichokes, include them in the layers. Top with a sprinkle of nutritional yeast, dairy-free cheese, herbs, and red pepper flakes if using.

Bake for 20 minutes.

Pesto Pasta

Pesto is one of summer's perfect foods. You can toss it over pasta, smear it on bread, or use it as a vegetable dip. Chef Alex Bury's recipe calls for basil, but you can use cilantro, basil, arugula, or a mix of your favorite herbs. The secret ingredient here is beans, which add creaminess and a protein kick. Walnuts or cashews can be used in place of the pine nuts, which are a little more expensive. Pesto keeps very well and is delicious the next day. It freezes well, too.

SERVES 4
TIME: 25 minutes

1 16-ounce package of your favorite pasta

2 cups tightly packed fresh basil leaves, washed and stems removed

2 cloves garlic, peeled

1 cup (½ of 15-ounce can) cooked navy beans or chickpeas, drained and rinsed

¼ cup raw walnuts or pine nuts

4 to 6 tablespoons extra virgin olive oil

3 tablespoons nutritional yeast

2 tablespoons lemon juice

2 teaspoons salt

Cook the pasta according to package directions.

Meanwhile, combine all other ingredients in a food processor with the "S" blade or using a high-power blender.

Process until smooth.

Taste and adjust the salt and lemon juice, as needed.

Toss over pasta.

PRO-TIP: Refrigerate in a covered container and use over the next 4 to 5 days. It also freezes well. Use as a spread on vegetable paninis or wraps, as a dip for vegetables, or as a sauce for meatless chicken. Add more oil or some water if you want it thinner (for tossing with pasta), or more beans if you want it thicker (for sandwich spreads).

Quick and Easy Pasta Marinara

Who needs store-bought sauce when you can whip up your own in just 20 minutes? You can use fresh herbs for added flavor if you have them on hand. Chef Alex Bury suggests serving atop your favorite pasta, as a dipping sauce for breadsticks, or in lasagna.

SERVES 4
TIME: 20 minutes

1 16-ounce package of your favorite pasta
½ cup yellow, red, or white onion, diced
¼ cup red wine or water
1 tablespoon garlic, minced
1 teaspoon dried basil, or 1 tablespoon fresh, chopped

1 teaspoon dried oregano, or 1 tablespoon fresh, chopped
1 teaspoon salt
⅛ teaspoon freshly ground black pepper
1 28-ounce can crushed tomatoes in juice
1 tablespoon balsamic vinegar

Cook the pasta according to package instructions.

In a medium saucepan, sauté the onion in the wine or water for 3 minutes to soften.

Add the garlic and sauté an additional 1 to 2 minutes, stirring constantly, or until fragrant but not browned. Add the herbs, salt, and pepper and sauté an additional 30 seconds.

Add the crushed tomatoes, including the juice, and the balsamic vinegar, stir well to combine, reduce the heat to low, and simmer the mixture for 10 minutes to blend the flavors.

Use right away, or allow it to cool and then store it in the refrigerator for up to one week, or freeze for up to two months.

Tuscan Pasta with White Beans, Asparagus, and Tomatoes

Pasta and beans is a traditional Italian combo with the filling goodness complemented with tangy tomatoes. You can throw in a handful of spinach or steamed broccoli florets to add a splash of color, or enjoy just it as is for an easy, delicious weeknight dinner. Get fancy and serve it with a big salad and a loaf of Italian bread for a date night.

SERVES 2
TIME: 20 minutes

8 ounces (half a package) of your favorite pasta
1 tablespoon extra virgin olive oil
3 cloves garlic, minced
½ onion, diced
1 15-ounce can diced tomatoes in juice
1 15-ounce can Great Northern or cannellini beans, drained and rinsed
1 teaspoon salt
1 tablespoon crushed red pepper flakes, optional
3 tablespoons chopped black olives, optional
½ bunch asparagus, chopped into thirds
½ bunch fresh parsley leaves, chopped
Chopped basil or oregano for garnish

Prepare the pasta according to package instructions.

In a medium saucepan, sauté the onion in the olive oil on medium for about 3 minutes or until translucent. Add the garlic and sauté for 2 minutes more. Add the tomatoes, including the juice, and bring to a simmer. Add the beans, salt, olives, and pepper, if using, and simmer for 10 minutes.

Stir in the asparagus and parsley and cook for 3 to 5 minutes or until the asparagus is bright green.

Toss sauce over pasta and serve. Garnish with chopped basil or oregano.

DIY Sushi

I travel a lot for work and have found that sushi is always a good meatless option on the road. I've had avocado rolls from Jackson, Mississippi, to Vancouver, Washington, and dozens of cities in between, and I've never been let down. But sushi's not only great for dining out: you can also make it at home.

When you're making your own, you can have fun and get creative. I've listed lots of filling options below, but the possibilities are endless—try shiitake mushrooms, cooked sweet potatoes, lightly steamed asparagus, or green beans—get crazy!

> **PRO-TIP:** Although rolling your own sushi may sound intimidating, it's actually quite easy. You can purchase a bamboo roller at an Asian market or in the cooking section of most department stores, but it's not necessary. Just keep your surface dry, be sure not to overstuff the rolls, and once you've rolled them, use a very sharp knife to cut them.

SERVES 2
TIME: 40 minutes

Sushi Rice
2 cups short grain sushi rice or other
   short grain rice

4 cups water
1 tablespoon sugar
1 tablespoon rice vinegar

Prepare the rice in a rice maker according to the manufacturer's instructions or add rice and water to a pot, bring to a boil, and then simmer for about 35 minutes until the water has completely evaporated. By this time, the rice should be very sticky. Remove from heat.

Mix together sugar and vinegar in a small bowl and stir into the rice, being careful not to make the rice mushy. Allow to cool until you can handle it.

(Continues)

(*Continued*)

Sushi

3 cups prepared sushi rice

4 to 6 sheets roasted nori

Your choice of vegetables:

½ avocado, cut lengthwise into strips

½ cucumber, cut lengthwise into strips

⅓ kabocha squash, peeled, cut into strips, and boiled for 15 minutes until tender

1 carrot, cut into thin strips, steamed for 5 minutes

3 leaves kale, stem removed, cut in half lengthwise, steamed for 5 minutes

1 jalapeño pepper, cut lengthwise into matchsticks

Once your rice is cool enough to handle, lay the nori on a dry surface, spread a handful of rice (a little goes a long way) along the bottom two-thirds of the nori. Line your vegetables up about 1 inch from the bottom of the nori lengthwise and roll into a log shape. Starting in the middle of the row, cut into sixths, about 1 inch per section. I use a serrated bread knife or steak knife as the nori can be tough to cut through without ruining the rolls.

Serve with soy sauce, wasabi, and pickled ginger.

Noodles with Peanut Sauce

This is a go-to recipe in my house for when I'm in a hurry to make dinner but want a meal that'll fill me up and also provide plenty of nutrients. Nutty peanut butter and salty soy sauce combine with a little sweetness plus hot sauce for an explosion of flavor. Packed with protein and ridiculously easy, this dish is a hit with kids for the taste and with parents for its ease. Adjust the spice as your family likes it.

SERVES 4
TIME: 15 minutes

Sauce
1 cup peanut butter
4 tablespoons soy sauce or tamari
2 teaspoons agave or other sweetener
1 teaspoon hot pepper sauce like sriracha, or more or less to taste
2 cloves garlic
1 to 1½ cups water
2 teaspoons toasted sesame oil

Vegetables
4 carrots, chopped into coins
2 cups broccoli florets
2 cups frozen edamame
Crushed peanuts or sesame seeds to garnish, optional
1 16-ounce package of your favorite noodles, cooked according to package instructions (spaghetti, angel hair, soba, and udon all work well)

Add all sauce ingredients to a blender or food processor, or use an immersion blender to combine well. If you like a thick sauce, use less water. Set aside.

Steam carrots, broccoli, and edamame for 4 minutes or until the broccoli is bright green.

Toss the vegetables with the noodles and pour the peanut sauce over it. Serve sprinkled with crushed peanuts or sesame seeds.

Steakless Pepper Steak

One of my favorite dishes my mom made when I was a kid was pepper steak. It was definitely not authentic, but it still had a wonderful flavor of caramelized onions and peppers swimming in a savory gravy that I love today. Back then I used to ask her to make pepper steak—without the steak. These days I make my own version, using her recipe, with a few modifications. It's fast, easy, and delicious and still one of my favorites.

SERVES 4
TIME: 25 minutes

2 tablespoons extra virgin olive oil
½ medium onion, sliced into half moons
1 large green or red bell pepper or
　2 medium, sliced (or a combo for
　more color)
1 jalapeño pepper, sliced, optional
1 15-ounce can diced tomatoes in juice

1 9-ounce package Gardein Beefless
　Tips, MorningStar Steak Strips,
　or braised tempeh (page 175)
1 tablespoon cornstarch
2 tablespoons soy sauce or tamari
Sesame seeds for garnish

Add the oil and onions to a large skillet and cook over medium heat. Sauté the onions for about 3 minutes until they begin to turn translucent. Add the peppers and cook for an additional 2 minutes.

Add the can of tomatoes, including the juice and allow to simmer for about 10 minutes. Add the beefless tips and cook until warmed through, about 5 minutes.

In a small bowl, combine the cornstarch with the soy sauce or tamari and mix until there are no lumps. Add to the skillet and mix in, stirring continuously until the sauce thickens. Serve over rice and give thanks to my mom for the delicious recipe.

Sprinkle with sesame seeds for extra flair.

Spicy Orange and Vegetarian Beef Stir-Fry with Broccoli

This is a very satisfying winter dish. With seasonal oranges in abundance, you can use some to dress up a classic combination. The zesty orange combines with spicy red peppers and a hint of sweetness to provide a flavorful sauce for juicy beefless tips.

SERVES 4
TIME: 30 minutes

3 oranges
3 tablespoons soy sauce or tamari
1 tablespoon rice wine
1 tablespoon cornstarch
½ teaspoon agave nectar
2 teaspoons extra virgin oil, divided
2 tablespoons minced garlic
2 tablespoons grated fresh ginger
3 to 4 small dried red chiles

1 package Gardein Beefless Tips, MorningStar Steak Strips, or baked tofu (page 173)
3 cups broccoli, cut into small florets
⅓ cup water
1 red bell pepper, seeded and sliced
¼ cup sliced scallion greens
Steamed rice

With a small sharp knife or vegetable peeler, carefully pare wide strips of zest from one of the oranges. Cut the zest into 1-inch pieces and set aside. Squeeze juice from the oranges into a small bowl (to make about ¾ cup). Add the soy sauce or tamari, rice wine, cornstarch, and agave and stir to combine; set aside.

Add the oil to the pan and heat until very hot. Carefully add the garlic, ginger, chiles, and the reserved orange zest; stir-fry until fragrant, about 30 seconds. Add the beefless tips, broccoli, and water. Cover and steam, stirring occasionally, until the water has evaporated and the broccoli sizzles, about 3 minutes. Add the bell pepper and stir-fry for 1 minute more.

Stir the reserved orange sauce and pour it into the pan. Bring to a boil, stirring, and cook until the sauce has thickened slightly, 1 to 2 minutes. Add scallion greens and toss to coat with sauce.

Serve over steamed rice.

Twenty-Minute Two-Bean Chili

G reat for cold days, this protein-packed chili is delicious, filling, and easy. It's called two-bean chili, but if you're feeling adventurous, add a third! The meat crumbles are optional; you can also add crumbled, braised tempeh (page 175), steel-cut oats cooked al dente—or go full bean! Serve with a side of warm maple corn muffins (page 159).

SERVES 2
TIME: 20 minutes of course!

2¼ cups water, divided
½ medium yellow onion, diced
2 cloves garlic, minced
1 jalapeño pepper, seeds removed and diced, optional
1 teaspoon chili powder
1 teaspoon ground cumin
1 teaspoon cayenne pepper, optional
1 teaspoon salt

1 15-ounce can diced tomatoes in juice
1 15-ounce can black beans, rinsed
1 15-ounce can red kidney beans, rinsed
1 cup meatless beef crumbles, optional (Beyond Meat, Yves, LightLife, or MorningStar)
Dairy-free sour cream or cheese for garnish

In a large nonstick saucepan, heat ¼ cup water over medium heat. Add the onion and sauté until translucent, about 3 minutes. Add the garlic and jalapeño pepper, if using, and sauté another 3 minutes, adding a splash of water if necessary to prevent sticking. Add the chili powder, cumin, cayenne if using, and salt. Cook for another 2 minutes.

Add 2 cups water, tomatoes and juice, and beans. Bring the mixture to a boil. Cover and simmer for 5 minutes. Add the beef crumbles, if using, and simmer for 5 more minutes.

Serve topped with a dollop of dairy-free sour cream or sprinkle of dairy-free cheese.

Macaroni and Cheese Surprise

W ho doesn't love a good macaroni and cheese? It's the quintessen- tial comfort food. This macaroni and cashew cheese doesn't have the same neon orange color of the food of my childhood, but it's much more delicious. The surprise is that not only is it tasty and comforting, but it's also healthy, with cashews offering the creaminess of cheese. You can use whatever vegetables you have on hand, but bright green broccoli makes a nice contrast. I eat this as a main course, but it can also be served as a side to baked tofu (page 173) and topped with Tennessee barbecue sauce (page 172).

SERVES 4
TIME: 20 minutes

1 pound of your favorite pasta (macaroni or shells work great)

1 head broccoli, cauliflower, or your favorite vegetable, cut into florets or small pieces

Cheese Sauce

1¼ cups raw cashews (if you have time to prepare in advance, soak them for an hour to overnight for a creamier sauce)

¼ cup nutritional yeast

1 teaspoon onion powder

1 teaspoon sea salt

½ teaspoon garlic powder

1½ cups plain, unsweetened soy or almond milk

¼ cup extra virgin olive oil

⅛ cup yellow miso

1 tablespoon lemon juice

¼ teaspoon paprika

Crushed walnuts or panko breadcrumbs, optional

Preheat oven to 350°F.

Prepare the pasta according to the package instructions. When 5 min- utes remain in the cook time, add in broccoli, cauliflower, or other vegeta- bles. Drain, rinse, and pour into a casserole dish. Set aside.

Meanwhile grind the cashews into a powder in a high-speed blender or food processor. Add the nutritional yeast, onion powder, salt, and garlic powder and blend thoroughly.

Add the soy or almond milk, oil, miso, and lemon juice and blend until smooth, scraping the sides to ensure they're thoroughly combined.

Toss the cheese sauce over the pasta and veggies and sprinkle with paprika. Bake for 20 minutes.

PRO-TIP: Crumble crushed walnuts or panko breadcrumbs over the top before baking for a fancier mac.

Old-Fashioned Chicken and Dumplings

This classic comfort dish of thick, warm broth with doughy dumplings gets a healthy boost with the addition of some vegetables. Decades ago, before it became common for us to eat meat at breakfast, lunch, and dinner, meat was stretched throughout a family's meals as in this recipe where it was traditionally used to add flavor to the stew. It's so flavorful, and the drop dumplings are surprisingly simple.

SERVES 4 to 6
TIME: 40 minutes

Dumplings
2 cups all-purpose flour or a 60/40 blend of all-purpose and whole wheat flours
1 tablespoon baking powder
½ teaspoon salt
½ stick (4 tablespoons) dairy-free margarine, like Earth Balance
¾ cup unsweetened plain soy or almond milk

Soup
1 tablespoon extra virgin olive oil
½ cup yellow or white onion, diced
2 stalks celery, chopped
8 ounces frozen mixed vegetables (half a bag)

½ cup all-purpose flour
½ teaspoon salt
1 teaspoon ground sage
½ teaspoon black pepper
8 cups vegetarian "no" chicken or vegetable broth (opt for the low-sodium variety or reduce salt in soup recipe)
1 cup meatless chicken, diced (Gardein Chick'n Scallopini, Beyond Meat Beyond Chicken strips, or MorningStar Farms Meal Starters Chik'n Strips)

To make the dumplings, combine the dry ingredients in a bowl.

Using a fork, cut the margarine in with the dry mixture until crumbly. Add the milk, stirring until moistened. Add more milk, 1 tablespoon at a time, if the mixture is too dry.

Knead the dough for 30 seconds, then pinch and roll into ½-inch balls. Set aside.

Meanwhile, in a large stockpot over medium heat sauté the onion and celery in the oil until the onion is translucent, about 3 minutes.

Add the frozen vegetables and cook until soft, about 4 minutes.

Add the flour, salt, sage, and pepper to make a thick paste. Slowly mix in the broth and bring to a boil.

Add the meatless chicken, and then drop in the dumplings one at a time, stirring gently. Reduce the heat and simmer for 20 minutes, stirring often.

If you'd like a thicker broth, in a separate bowl combine 2 tablespoons flour with 3 tablespoons water, mix vigorously, and add to broth.

Serve hot.

Classic Chicken-Free Pot Pie

On rainy days when you want to curl up in bed with the covers up to your chin and a good book, this pot pie will warm your home and your soul. Loaded with vegetables in creamy, savory gravy and enveloped by a flaky, warm crust, it will satisfy you from your taste buds to your belly.

SERVES 4
TIME: 50 minutes; 25 minutes active

2 unbaked piecrusts
1 tablespoon extra virgin olive oil
½ yellow onion, diced
1 clove garlic, minced
2 white potatoes, cubed
¼ cup water
8 ounces mixed frozen vegetables,
    containing peas, corn, carrots,
    green beans

1 cup meatless chicken, cut into ½ inch
    cubes (Gardein Chick'n Scallopini,
    MorningStar Chick'n Strips, Beyond
    Meat all work well)
2 cups gravy, see recipe below

Preheat oven to 375°F. In a large saucepan over medium heat, sauté the onion in the oil until translucent, about 3 minutes. Add the garlic and potatoes and ¼ cup water, and cook for 10 minutes until potatoes are just slightly tender, yet firm. Add the frozen vegetables and chicken, and cook for 3 to 5 minutes.

Meanwhile, make the gravy (recipe below).

Pour the gravy over the vegetable-and-chicken mixture and stir. Pour into one pie shell. Place another shell on top of the pie. Use a fork to press down and seal the edges, and then use a fork or knife to poke a few holes in the top of pie to allow air to escape. Bake for 25 to 30 minutes. Allow to cool for 10 minutes before serving.

Gravy

2 tablespoons extra virgin olive oil
2 tablespoons all-purpose or whole wheat
    flour or a mixture of the two
2 tablespoons nutritional yeast
2 cups low sodium vegetable broth or
    2 cups water plus low sodium bouillon
    paste sufficient to make 2 cups per
    package instructions

½ teaspoon dried powdered sage,
    optional
¼ teaspoon black pepper, more to taste
Sage
Pinch of salt, to taste

In a large skillet, toast the flour and nutritional yeast in olive oil on medium heat for 2 minutes or until it starts to brown.

Lower heat and slowly add the broth, stirring and using a fork to crush any lumps that may form. Add the pepper, sage, and salt, if using. Return heat to medium until the gravy begins to bubble and thicken.

Allow to simmer for 3 to 5 minutes, stirring regularly.

Cuban Rice and Beans

This recipe is the ideal weeknight dish. It's easy, filling, and delicious, and it's also very affordable. The cumin and salsa combine to create savory Cuban flavors. Chef Alex suggests topping with sliced avocado or guacamole. Or for a kid-friendly meal, use corn chips as scoopers.

SERVES 4
TIME: 40 minutes; 10 minutes active

2 cups cooked rice, white or brown
½ cup finely diced mild red, yellow, or white onion
1 tablespoon extra virgin olive oil
2 cloves garlic, minced
1 cup salsa (spice level to taste)
1 teaspoon cumin

1 4-ounce can diced green chiles or ¼ cup diced fresh, or more salsa
½ cup chopped scallions (green onions), including green portion, optional
1 15-ounce can black beans, drained, or 2 cups cooked, drained

Cook rice according to the package instructions.

Meanwhile in a medium pan, sauté the onions in oil on medium heat until translucent, about 3 minutes. Add the garlic and sauté 2 minutes more. Remove from heat.

Once the rice is fully cooked, in a medium bowl, toss all ingredients together. Serve and enjoy!

Hoppin' John

Hoppin' John is a Southern stew of black-eyed peas and rice. It's traditionally eaten on New Year's Day to ensure a prosperous forthcoming year. The black-eyed peas are emblematic of coins, which is apt, as they're an inexpensive source of protein. Chef Alex skips the customary ham hock here in favor of liquid smoke, which provides a smoky, rich flavor. Enjoy Hoppin' John any time of the year, doused in hot sauce!

SERVES 4
TIME: 45 minutes; 25 minutes active

2 cups cooked rice, white or brown
1 tablespoon extra virgin olive oil
1 cup onion, chopped
¼ cup celery, chopped
½ cup green bell pepper, chopped
2 cloves garlic, minced
1 pound black-eyed peas, soaked
    overnight and rinsed
1 quart low sodium vegetable broth
    or 1 quart water plus low sodium
    bouillon paste sufficient to make
    1 quart per package instructions

1 bay leaf
1 teaspoon dry thyme leaves
1 teaspoon cumin
½ teaspoon liquid smoke, optional
1 tablespoon soy sauce or tamari
8 ounces chopped tempeh bacon or
    Tofurky Andouille sausage, optional

In a large pot, sauté the onion, celery, pepper, and garlic in the oil for 1 minute over medium heat.

Add the black-eyed peas, stock, and bay leaf. Bring to a boil, then reduce to a simmer and cook for 20 minutes.

Add the rest of the seasonings and cook for another 20 to 30 minutes, until the peas are tender. Add more water if needed to ensure the mixture doesn't dry out.

Remove the bay leaf.

Serve hot over freshly cooked rice. Garnish with tempeh bacon or Tofurky sausage, if using.

ALTERNATIVE METHOD: You can also use 2 cans of cooked black-eyed peas. Add the seasonings above (but not the stock) and heat until warmed through.

Simple Southwestern Burrito Roll Ups

C hef Alex's burrito roll ups are a great recipe to make with kids. They can safely help spread the beans and salsa and help divide the beans so there's an equal amount for each tortilla. And of course they love rolling them up! You don't have to ruin the fun by telling them the burritos are good for them, but you can take comfort in knowing so.

SERVES 4 to 6
TIME: 10 minutes

1 10-count package large flour tortillas
1 jar of your favorite salsa
1 15-ounce can fat-free refried beans

Optional additions:
Meatless chicken strips, ground beef,
    or soyrizo

Sautéed spinach
Your favorite dairy-free cheese
Cooked rice
Sautéed vegetables (mushrooms, onions,
    and peppers)

Preheat oven to 350ºF. Spread each tortilla with a thin layer of beans.

Add 2 to 3 spoonfuls of the salsa, and spread it out over the beans. Add additions, if using.

Roll up like a cigar.

Place all the wraps on a cookie sheet and bake for 10 minutes until the outside of the wraps are slightly brown and crispy.

Desserts

Mocha Rice Pudding

C hef Alex Bury loves coffee in any form and swears by this recipe, but you don't have to love coffee to love this dessert. Dark chocolate and coffee provide a depth of flavor that perfectly balances out the sweetness. Serve it warm on cold winter nights. Serve it cold as a way to beat the heat.

SERVES 4
TIME: 1 hour

¾ cup long grain white rice
5 cups unsweetened plain soy or
   almond milk
1 cup strong brewed coffee
4 to 6 tablespoons maple syrup
   or 4 to 6 chopped pitted dates

Pinch of salt
Dash of cinnamon
½ cup dairy-free dark chocolate chips
1 tablespoon vanilla
Chopped almonds, chocolate shavings, or
   a sprinkle of cinnamon for garnish

Combine the rice, soy or almond milk, coffee, maple syrup or dates, salt, and cinnamon in a heavy sauce pan.

Bring to a boil, and then simmer (uncovered) for at least 45 minutes, stirring often.

When the rice is very soft and creamy, stir in the chocolate and vanilla, and then turn off the heat.

Serve warm or chilled. Top with chopped almonds, chocolate shavings, or a sprinkle of cinnamon.

Chocolate Pecan Pie

How can you make pecan pie even better? Add chocolate. Chef Alex Bury's Chocolate Pecan Pie is an easy and delicious recipe to impress your family at a holiday dinner.

SERVES 6 to 8
TIME: 45 minutes, plus 6 hours' cooling time

1 cup maple syrup
2 cups pecans
1 tablespoon vanilla extract
¼ teaspoon salt
2 tablespoons arrowroot powder
⅓ cup unsweetened plain soy or
    almond milk

1 cup dairy-free dark chocolate chips,
    melted
1 pre-made whole wheat, vegan pie crust
    (found in freezer sections) or make
    your own

Preheat oven to 350°F.

Stir the maple syrup, pecans, vanilla, and salt together.

In a separate bowl, whisk together the arrowroot and soy or almond milk. Add to the maple syrup mixture.

Whisk in the melted chocolate.

Pour into unbaked pie shell and bake for about 30 minutes, until the crust is golden brown.

Allow to cool before serving. It will firm up, but it needs about 6 hours to do that.

Summer Peach Cobbler

This easy dessert takes me back to my childhood summers at Grandma's house. Buttery and decadent, you won't believe how simple it is. Although peaches are my go-to cobbler filling, you could swap them out for apples and cinnamon, blueberries, blackberries, or even pitted sour cherries.

SERVES 6 to 8
TIME: 1 hour, 15 minutes; 15 minutes active

8 tablespoons (1 stick) dairy-free margarine, like Earth Balance, melted

1 cup all-purpose flour

1½ teaspoons baking powder

¼ teaspoon salt

1 cup granulated sugar

1 cup unsweetened plain soy or almond milk

2 cups fresh sliced peaches (frozen and thawed, or fresh peaches, berries, apples—whatever you prefer)

Preheat oven to 350ºF. I generally put the margarine in a large casserole dish and stick it in the oven to melt while the oven preheats.

In a medium bowl, mix the flour, baking powder, salt, and sugar. Add the soy or almond milk and mix together with a whisk.

Carefully remove the casserole dish from the oven and pour the batter over the melted margarine. Pour the fruit over the mixture.

Bake for 1 hour until the top is golden brown and the crust has risen over the fruit. It's best when served warm (with a scoop of vanilla dairy-free ice cream).

Pineapple Upside-Down Cake

C hef Alex Bury's spin on this classic dessert is buttery, rich, and flavorful, yet it comes without the fat of conventional recipes. The flavor of pineapple provides a taste of the tropics while the fruit keeps the cake spongy and moist. This makes a delicious and beautiful dessert to bring along to a summer picnic or potluck.

SERVES 8 to 10
TIME: 55 minutes; 10 minutes active

¼ cup agave nectar

1 tablespoon lemon juice

1 pineapple, cut into chunks or rings, or 1 20-ounce can unsweetened pineapple

1½ cups whole wheat pastry flour

2¼ teaspoons baking powder

½ teaspoon cinnamon

¼ teaspoon dried ginger

¼ teaspoon nutmeg

¼ teaspoon cloves

¼ teaspoon salt

1 cup unsweetened, plain soy or almond milk

½ cup maple syrup

1½ teaspoons vanilla

Preheat oven to 350ºF.

Lightly oil a 9-inch cake pan or use a nonstick pan. Drizzle the agave nectar and lemon juice over the bottom of the pan. Arrange the pineapple rings to cover the bottom of the pan.

In a medium bowl, mix the dry ingredients well. In a separate bowl, whisk together the wet ingredients. Make a well in the center of the dry ingredients, add the wet ingredients to the dry, mix well, and then pour over the fruit. Bake until a toothpick inserted into the center comes out clean, about 40 minutes. Allow to cool for 10 minutes and then invert onto a cooling rack or serving plate.

Royal Hot Fudge Sauce

Chef Alex's decadent, rich sauce is a perfect topping for cakes, desserts, and dairy-free ice cream, or as a dipping sauce for fruit. To top that off, it's ready in just 10 minutes!

MAKES 2 cups
TIME: 10 minutes

½ cup cocoa powder

2 teaspoons cornstarch

1¼ cups fat-free plain, unsweetened rice, soy, or almond milk

½ cup maple syrup

1 tablespoon vanilla extract

In a small bowl, sift together the cocoa and cornstarch.

Transfer the cocoa mixture to a small saucepan and whisk in ½ cup milk until smooth.

Add the remaining milk and maple syrup to the saucepan and whisk well to combine.

Cook the mixture over medium heat, while whisking constantly, for 2 to 3 minutes or until it forms a thick sauce.

Remove the saucepan from the heat and whisk in the vanilla.

Serve immediately or allow to cool and store in an airtight container in the refrigerator for up to two weeks, reheating as needed.

Notes

Introduction

1. "Pets By the Numbers: U.S. Pet Ownership, Community Cat and Shelter Population Estimates, 2012–2016," Humane Society of the United States, http://www.humanesociety.org/issues/pet overpopulation/facts/pet_ownership _statistics.html (n.d.).

2. "How Many Teens and Other Youth Are Vegetarian and Vegan? The Vegetarian Resource Groups Asks in a 2014 National Poll," Vegetarian Resource Group Blog, http://www.vrg.org/blog/2014/05/30/how-many-teens-and-other -youth-are-vegetarian-and-vegan-the-vegetarian-resource-group-asks-in-a -2014-national-poll/ (May 30, 2014).

3. Anne-Claire Vergnaud, et al., "Meat Consumption and Prospective Weight Change in Participants of the EPIC-PANACEA Study," *American Journal of Clinical Nutrition* 92 (2010): 398–407.

4. Philip J. Tuso, et al., "Nutritional Update for Physicians: Plant-Based Diets," *Permanente Journal* 17.2 (2013): 61–66.

5. Patricia Cobe, "2015's Top Menu Stories," *Foodservice Director*, http://www.foodservicedirector.com/menu-development/menu-strategies /articles/2015s-top-menu-stories (December 2015).

6. Ashley Pearson, "Is Going Vegan the Secret to a Body Like Jennifer Lopez's? Ashley Pearson Tries One of the Year's Most Popular Eating Crazes," *Daily Mail*, http://www.dailymail.co.uk/femail/article-2781948/Is-going-vegan -secret-body-like-Jennifer-Lopez-s-Ashley-Pearson-tries-one-year-s-popular -eating-crazes.htlm (October 7, 2014).

7. Brittany Brady, "New York School Goes All-Vegetarian," CNN, http://www.cnn.com/2013/05/02/health/new-york-vegetarian-school/ (May 2, 2013); and Eric Pfeiffer, "Sheriff Joe Arpaio Institutes Cost-Saving, Vegetarian Meals for Inmates," *Yahoo News*, http://news.yahoo.com/blogs/sideshow/sheriff -joe-arpaio-institutes-cost-saving--vegetarian-meals-for-inmates-220538735 .html (September 25, 2013).

Chapter 1: Eating Ourselves to Death

1. Eric O'Grey, op-ed written for *San Jose Mercury News*, unpublished (September 1, 2013).

2. Eric O'Grey, "Letter to President Clinton Sparks My First Interview," http://breaking4.blogspot.com/2012/12/letter-to-president-clinton-sparks -my.html (December 15, 2012).

3. Dawn Jackson Blatner, "Flexitarian FAQ," https://dawnjacksonblatner. com/books/the-flexitarian-diet/flexitarian-faq/ (accessed June 24, 2016); P. K. Newby, Katherine Tucker, et al., "Risk of Overweight and Obesity among Semivegetarian, Lactovegetarian, and Vegan Women," *American Journal of Clinical Nutrition* 81.6 (June 2005): 1267–1274; "The Flexitarian Diet," *US News and World Report*, http://health.usnews.com/best-diet/flexitarian-diet (accessed June 24, 2016).

4. Carina Storrs, "Americans Are Cutting Calories, But Far From Eating Healthy," CNN Health, http://www.cnn.com/2015/07/30/health/americans -cutting-calories/ (July 30, 2015); "News Release: American Adults are Choosing Healthier Foods, Consuming Healthier Diets," U.S. Department of Agriculture, http://www.usda.gov/wps/portal/usda/usdahome?content idonly=true&contentid=2014/01/0008.xml (January 16, 2014); Melinda Beck and Amy Schatz, "Americans' Eating Habits Take a Healthier Turn, Study Finds Working-Age Adults Consume Fewer Calories, Eat Out Less," *Wall Street Journal*, http://www.wsj.com/articles/SB10001424052702304149404579323092 916490748 (January 16, 2014); and Marygrace Taylor, "39% of Americans Are Eating Less Meat," *Prevention*, http://www.prevention.com/food/smart -shopping/39-americans-are-eating-less-meat (January 29, 2014).

5. "Leading Causes of Death," Centers for Disease Control and Prevention, from http://www.cdc.gov/nchs/fastats/leading-causes-of-death.htm (April 26, 2016).

6. "Heart Disease: Scope and Impact," Heart Disease Foundation, http://www.theheartfoundation.org/heart-disease-facts/heart-disease -statistics/ (n.d.).

7. Mayo Clinic staff, "Heart Disease," http://www.mayoclinic.org/diseases -conditions/heart-disease/basics/definition/con-20034056 (July 29, 2014).

8. "Congestive Heart Failure," University of Southern California Keck Medical School, http://www.cts.usc.edu/zglossary-congestiveheartfailure .html (n.d.).

9. Phil Hardesty, "Have Heart Disease? Feel Confident Resuming Sexual Activity!" http://ornishspectrum.com/video/heart-disease/ (2015).

10. W. C. Roberts, "It's the Cholesterol, Stupid!" *American Journal of Cardiology* 106 (2010): 1364–1366.

11. "About Cholesterol," American Heart Association, http://www.heart.org /HEARTORG/Conditions/Cholesterol/AboutCholesterol/About-Cholesterol _UCM_001220_Article.jsp (July 31, 2014).

12. "What Is Cholesterol?" National Institutes of Health, http://www.nhlbi .nih.gov/health/health-topics/topics/hbc/ (September 19, 2012).

13. "Kings of the Carnivores," *The Economist*, http://www.economist.com /blogs/graphicdetail/2012/04/daily-chart-17 (April 30, 2012).

14. Caldwell Esselstyn and Mladen Golubic, "The Nutritional Reversal of Cardiovascular Disease—Fact or Fiction? Three Case Reports," *Experimental & Clinical Cardiology* 20.7 (2014), http://www.dresselstyn.com/Esselstyn_Three -case-reports_Exp-Clin-Cardiol-July-2014.pdf.

15. "Adult Obesity Facts," Centers for Disease Control and Prevention, http://www.cdc.gov/obesity/data/adult.html (June 16, 2015).

16. Eric A. Finkelstein, et al., "Obesity and Severe Obesity Forecasts Through 2030," *American Journal of Preventative Medicine* 42.6 (June 2013): 563–570, http://www.ajpmonline.org/article/S0749-3797(12)00146-8/fulltext.

17. "Adult Obesity Facts," http://www.cdc.gov/obesity/data/adult.html.

18. Michael Greger, "Uprooting the Leading Causes of Death," NutritionFacts.org, http://nutritionfacts.org/video/uprooting-the-leading -causes-of-death/ (July 26, 2012).

19. Jeff Gordinier, "My Dinner With Longevity Expert Dan Buettner (No Kale Required)," *New York Times*, http://www.nytimes.com/2015/08/02 /fashion/dinner-with-blue-zones-solution-dan-buettner.html?_r=0 (August 2, 2015).

20. "News Release: Diets High in Meat Consumption Associated with Obesity," Johns Hopkins Bloomberg School of Public Health (September 3, 2009).

21. Anne-Claire Vergnaud, et al., "Meat Consumption and Prospective Weight Change in Participants of the EPIC-PANACEA Study," *American Journal of Clinical Nutrition* 92 (2010): 398–407.

22. "Vegetarian Diets," American Heart Association, http://www.heart.org /HEARTORG/GettingHealthy/NutritionCenter/Vegetarian-Diets_UCM _306032_Article.jsp (March 19, 2014).

23. "The Plant-Based Diet: A Healthier Way to Eat," Kaiser Permanente, http://mydoctor.kaiserpermanente.org/ncal/Images/New%20Plant%20Based %20Booklet%201214_tcm28-781815.pdf (2013).

24. Philip J. Tuso, et al., "Nutritional Update for Physicians: Plant-Based Diets," *Permanente Journal* 17.2 (Spring 2013): 61–66.

Chapter 2: A Tale of Two Chickens

1. J. L. Lusk, R. W. Norwood, and Prickett, "Consumer Preferences for Farm Animal Welfare: Results of a Nationwide Telephone Survey" (2007).

2. "Pets by the Numbers," Humane Society of the United States, http://www.humanesociety.org/issues/pet_overpopulation/facts/pet_ownership _statistics.html (January 30, 2014).

3. Brad Tuttle, "Psych Experts: There's Nothing Crazy About Giving Christmas Presents to Pets," *Time*, http://business.time.com/2011/12/20 /psych-experts-theres-nothing-crazy-about-giving-christmas-presents-to-pets / (December 20, 2011).

4. William Grimes, "If Chickens Are So Smart, Why Aren't They Eating Us?" *New York Times*, http://www.nytimes.com/2003/01/12/weekinreview/if -chickens-are-so-smart-why-aren-t-they-eating-us.html (January 12, 2003).

5. "Factory Farming: Chicken," Massachusetts SPCA, www.mspca.org /programs/animal-protection-legislation/animal-welfare/farm-animal-welfare /factory-farming/chicken/ (2014).

6. "Chickens Are Capable of Feeling Empathy, Scientists Believe," *The Telegraph*, http://www.telegraph.co.uk/science/science-news/8370301/Chickens -are-capable-of-feeling-empathy-scientists-believe.html (March 9, 2011).

7. Victoria Gill, "Baby Chicks Do Basic Arithmetic," BBC News, http://news.bbc.co.uk/2/hi/science/nature/7975260.stm (April 1, 2009).

8. "Glossary of Poultry Terms," University of Kentucky College of Food, Agriculture and Environment, http://afspoultry.ca.uky.edu/extension-glossary (July 5, 2015).

9. Carolynn Smith and Sarah Zielinski, "Brainy Bird," *Scientific American* (February 2014).

10. "About Chickens," Humane Society International, http://www.hsi.org /assets/pdfs/about_chickens.pdf (May 2014).

11. M. Follensbee, "Quantifying the Nesting Motivation of Hens," dissertation, University of Guelph, Ontario, Canada (1992).

12. "Mother Hen, definition," *Merriam Webster's Dictionary*, http://www .merriam-webster.com/dictionary/mother%20hen (2015).

13. "About Chickens," http://www.hsi.org/assets/pdfs/about_chickens.pdf.

14. Ibid.

15. "How to Read Meat and Dairy Labels," Humane Society of the United States, http://www.humanesociety.org/issues/confinement_farm/facts/meat _dairy_labels.html (n.d.).

16. Isabelle Cnudde, phone interview with the author (May 31, 2016).

17. "Scientists and Experts on Battery Cages and Laying Hen Welfare," Humane Society of the United States, http://www.humanesociety.org/assets /pdfs/farm/HSUS-Synopsis-of-Expert-Opinions-on-Battery-Cages-and -Hen-Welfare.pdf (n.d.).

18. "An HSUS Report: The Welfare of Animals in the Chicken Industry,"

Humane Society of the United States, http://www.humanesociety.org/assets
/pdfs/farm/welfare_broiler.pdf (2013).

19. Ibid.

20. "Pulmonary Arterial Hypertension (ascites syndrome)," University of
Arkansas (2013).

21. "An HSUS Report: The Welfare of Animals in the Chicken Industry,"
http://www.humanesociety.org/assets/pdfs/farm/welfare_broiler.pdf (n.d.).

22. Ibid.

23. "Unsafe at These Speeds," Southern Poverty Law Center, http://www
.splcenter.org/get-informed/publications/unsafe-at-these-speeds/worker-safety
-a-low-priority/chicken-catchers-face-grueling-dangerous-co (February 28,
2013).

24. Ibid.

25. "An HSUS Report: The Welfare of Animals in the Chicken Industry,"
http://www.humanesociety.org/assets/pdfs/farm/welfare_broiler.pdf.

26. Josh Balk, interview with the author (March 9, 2015).

27. Ibid.

28. 2010. "Can You Ask a Pig if His Glass Is Half Full?" *Science Daily*,
https://www.sciencedaily.com/releases/2010/07/100727201515.htm (July 28,
2010).

Chapter 3: It's Getting Hot in Here

1. Ben Peterson, personal interview with the author (July 29, 2015).

2. "Meat packing industry," Occupational Safety & Health Administration,
https://www.osha.gov/SLTC/meatpacking/ (n.d.).

3. Robbie Silverman, "No Relief for Poultry Workers," Oxfam America,
http://politicsofpoverty.oxfamamerica.org/2016/05/no-relief-for-poultry
-workers/ (May 11, 2016).

4. "No Relief: Denial of Bathroom Breaks in Poultry Industry," Oxfam
America, https://www.oxfamamerica.org/explore/research-publications/no
-relief/ (2016).

5. "Workplace Safety and Health: Safety in the Meat and Poultry Industry,
while Improving, Could Be Further Strengthened," U.S. Government
Accountability Office, http://www.gao.gov/new.items/d0596.pdf (January 2005).

6. Ibid.

7. Ibid.

8. "Butterball's House of Horrors: A PETA Undercover Investigation,"
People for the Ethical Treatment of Animals, http://www.peta.org/features
/butterball-peta-investigation/ (n.d.); and "Investigation Reveals Cruelty at
Pig Factory Farm," Mercy for Animals, http://pigs.mercyforanimals.org/ (n.d.).

9. Jason Dearen, "Residents Fight to Clean Up California Chicken Waste," *Associated Press/Capital Press*, http://www.capitalpress.com/content/AP-farm -scene-chicken-waste-021910 (March 4, 2010).

10. Tracie Cone, "Jury Says Central Calif. Chicken Egg Farm Is Foul," Associated Press, http://www.deseretnews.com/article/700138735/Jury-says -Central-Calif-chicken-egg-farm-is-foul.html (May 25, 2011).

11. "Chickens and the Egg," *San Francisco Bay Guardian*, http://www.sfbg .com/print/2008/10/29/chickens-and-egg (October 28, 2008).

12. Will Frampton, "Olivera Egg Ranch Stench Has French Camp Neighbors Angry, Suing," *ABC News 10*, KXTV, http://archive.news10.net /news/story.aspx?storyid=90869 (August 13, 2010).

13. Cone, "Jury Says Central Calif. Chicken Egg Farm Is Foul."

14. Nathan Pelletier and Peter Tyedmers, "Forecasting Potential Global Environmental Costs of Livestock Production 2000–2050," Proceedings of the National Academy of Sciences of the United States of America. 17 August. Available from http://www.pnas.org/content/107/43/18371.full.pdf (August 17, 2010).

15. A. Ertug Ercin, et al., "Ecological Indicators: The Water Footprint of Soy Milk and Soy Burger and Equivalent Animal Products," *Ecological Indicators,* 18 (December 11, 2011): 392–402.

16. Julia Lurie, "Here's What I Saw in a California Town Without Running Water," *Mother Jones*, http://www.motherjones.com/environment/2015/08 /drought-no-running-water-east-porterville (September 7, 2015).

17. Jessica Glenza, "The California Town with No Water: Even an 'Angel' Can't Stop the Wells Going Dry," *The Guardian*, http://www.theguardian.com /us-news/2015/apr/20/east-porterville-california-drought-bottled-water -showers-toilets (April 20, 2015).

18. Ibid.

19. Lurie, "Here's What I Saw in a California Town Without Running Water."

20. "State Water Project Allocation Increased," California Department of Water Resources, http://water.ca.gov/waterconditions/ (April 21, 2016).

21. Julian Fulton, et al., "California's Water Footprint," *Pacific Institute*, http://pacinst.org/app/uploads/2013/02/ca_ftprint_full_report3.pdf (December 2012); and D. L. Marrin, "Reducing Water and Energy Footprints Via Dietary Changes among Consumers," *International Journal of Nutrition and Food Sciences* 3.5 (August 20, 2014): 361–369.

22. David Pimentel and Marcia Pimentel, "Sustainability of Meat-Based and Plant-Based Diets and the Environment," *American Journal of Clinical Nutrition* 78 (suppl, 2003): 660S–663S, http://ajcn.nutrition.org/content/78/3/660S.full.

23. "Blue Lunchbox Challenge," One Drop, http://www.onedrop.org/calcul/pdf/BLUE%20LUNCHBOX_challenge.pdf (2015).

24. Jennie Saxe, "Water with Your Meal?" Environmental Protection Agency, https://blog.epa.gov/blog/2016/02/water-with-your-meal/ (February 25, 2016).

25. "Soy Milk," Water Footprint Network, http://waterprint.net/soy_milk.html (n.d.).

26. A. Ertug Ercin, et al., "Ecological Indicators: The Water Footprint of Soy Milk and Soy Burger and Equivalent Animal Products."

27. Mesfin Mekonnen and Arjen Hoekstra, "A Global Assessment of the Water Footprint of Farm Animal Products," 24 January. *Ecosystems* 15.3 (January 24, 2012): 401–415, http://waterfootprint.org/media/downloads/Mekonnen-Hoekstra-2012-WaterFootprintFarmAnimalProducts.pdf.

28. Kenneth Mathews and Rachel Johnson, "Alternative Beef Production Systems: Issues and Implications," Economic Research Service of the USDA, http://www.ers.usda.gov/media/1071057/ldpm-218-01.pdf (April 2013).

29. Kenneth Mathews, "Cattle and Beef Background," Economic Research Service of the USDA, http://www.ers.usda.gov/topics/animal-products/cattle-beef/background.aspx (May 13, 2016).

30. "Corn," Water Footprint Network, http://waterprint.net/corn.html (n.d.).

31. "California Drought: Livestock, Dairy, and Poultry Sectors," U.S. Department of Agriculture, Economic Research Service, http://www.ers.usda.gov/topics/in-the-news/california-drought-farm-and-food-impacts/california-drought-livestock,-dairy,-and-poultry-sectors.aspx (June 25, 2015).

32. Brianna Sacks, "California Dairy Farmers Struggling to Survive Prolonged Drought," *Los Angeles Times*, http://www.latimes.com/business/la-fi-drought-dairy-20141003-story.html (October 3, 2014).

33. Robbin Marks, "Cesspools of Shame: How Factory Farm Lagoons and Sprayfields Threaten Environmental and Public Health," Natural Resources Defense Council and the Clean Water Network, http://www.nrdc.org/water/pollution/cesspools/cesspools.pdf (2001).

34. Sara Peach, "What to Do About Pig Poop? North Carolina Fights a Rising Tide," *National Geographic*, http://news.nationalgeographic.com/news/2014/10/141028-hog-farms-waste-pollution-methane-north-carolina-environment/ (October 30, 2014).

35. Arelis R. Hernandez, et al., "Factory farming practices are under scrutiny again in N.C. after disastrous hurricane floods," *Washington Post*, https://www.washingtonpost.com/news/capital-weather-gang/wp/2016/10/16/factory-farming-practices-are-under-scrutiny-again-in-n-c-after-disastrous-hurricane-floods/ (October 16, 2016).

36. Rebecca Leung, "Pork Power: Are Hog Farmers Creating A Waste Hazard?" *60 Minutes: CBS News*, http://www.cbsnews.com/news/pork-power / (June 19, 2003).

37. Peter T. Kilborn, "Hurricane Reveals Flaws in Farm Law as Animal Waste Threatens N. Carolina Water," *New York Times*, http://www.nytimes .com/1999/10/17/us/hurricane-reveals-flaws-in-farm-law-as-animal-waste -threatens-n-carolina-water.html?src=pm&pagewanted=2 (October 17, 1999).

38. "NC Aquatic Dead zone from floods after Hurricane Floyd," McGraw Hill, http://www.mhhe.com/biosci/pae/es_map/articles/article_53.mhtml (October 1999); and Estes Thompson, "Floyd's Runoff Creates 'Dead Zone' Off North Carolina," *Southcoast Today*, http://www.southcoasttoday.com/apps/pbcs.dll /article?AID=/19991009/NEWS/310099983&cid=sitesearch (January 11, 2011).

39. MacKenzie Elmer, "Spills Trigger Second, Third Fish Kill in Iowa This Week," *Des Moines Register*, http://www.desmoinesregister.com/story/news /crime-and-courts/2015/10/01/spills-trigger-second-third-fish-kill-iowa -week/73138172/ (October 1, 2015).

40. "2015 Gulf of Mexico Dead Zone 'Above Average,'" National Oceanic and Atmospheric Administration, http://www.noaanews.noaa.gov/stories 2015/080415-gulf-of-mexico-dead-zone-above-average.html (August 2015).

41. "Hypoxia in the Gulf of Mexico: a Growing Problem," Institute for Agriculture and Trade Policy, http://www.iatp.org/files/Hypoxia_in_the_Gulf _of_Mexico_A_growing_proble.pdf (2002).

42. Joby Warrick, "Large 'Dead Zone' Signals More Problems for Chesapeake Bay," *Washington Post*, https://www.washingtonpost.com/national/health-science /large-dead-zone-signals-continued-problems-for-the-chesapeake-bay/2014 /08/31/1e0c2024-2fc2-11e4-9b98-848790384093_story.html (August 31, 2014).

43. "Facts about Maryland's Meat Chicken Industry," Delmarva Poultry Industry, https://www.dpichicken.org/faq_facts/docs/factsmd2014.pdf (2015).

44. Rudi Keller, "Hog Waste Spill in Callaway Raises Concerns about CAFO Plans," *Columbia Tribune*, http://www.columbiatribune.com/news/local/hog -waste-spill-in-callaway-raises-concerns-about-cafo-plans/article_7c2f043e -9227-5481-a8bb-14bef64b5a7e.html (2014).

45. "Clean up and Abatement Order," California Regional Water Quality Control Board Central Valley Region, http://www.waterboards.ca.gov/central valley/board_decisions/adopted_orders/stanislaus/r5-2014-0701_cao.pdf (2014).

46. Michael Wines, "Behind Toledo's Water Crisis, a Long-Troubled Lake Erie," *New York Times*, http://www.nytimes.com/2014/08/05/us/lifting-ban -toledo-says-its-water-is-safe-to-drink-again.html?_r=3 (August 4, 2014).

47. Sarah Peach, "What to Do About Pig Poop? North Carolina Fights a Rising Tide," *National Geographic*, http://news.nationalgeographic.com/news

/2014/10/141028-hog-farms-waste-pollution-methane-north-carolina
-environment/ (October 30, 2014).

48. Lee Bergquist, "Farmer's Past Pollution Cited By Opponents of
New Dairy Farm," *Milwaukee Journal Sentinel*, http://www.jsonline.com
/news/wisconsin/proposed-dairy-farm-raises-pollution-concerns-b99245524
z1-254971321.html (April 13, 2014); and "Adam's Heifer-Raising Farm to Pay
Fine for Water Pollution," Madison.com, http://host.madison.com/news/local
/crime_and_courts/adams-heifer-raising-farm-to-pay-fine-for-water-pollution
/article_ca093561-c320-5691-a579-4a468cf925e7.html (August 30, 2013).

49. Garret Ellison, "Liquid Manure Spill from Allegan County Farm
Threatening Rabbit River, Says DEQ," MLive.com, http://www.mlive.com
/news/grand-rapids/index.ssf/2014/02/schaendorf_farm_manure_spill.html
(February 16, 2014).

50. "1 Million-Gallon Manure Spill Fouls Root River in Minnesota,"
Associated Press, *Lacrosse Tribune*, http://lacrossetribune.com/news/local/millon
-gallon-manure-spill-fouls-root-river-in-minnesota/article_1d32bf50-a715
-11e2-b4ac-001a4bcf887a.html (April 17, 2013).

51. "News Release: Dairy Company Owner Sentenced to Six Months of
Home Detention and Ordered to Pay $15,000 Fine for Discharging 11,000
Gallons of Cow Feces into the French Broad River," Environmental Protection
Agency, https://yosemite.epa.gov/opa/admpress. nsf/21b8983ffa5d0e4685257
dd4006b85e2/8faa35ddc66eaa9a85257e380055b9fb!OpenDocument (May 1,
2015).

52. "Illinois Hog Farm Will Pay Fines Over Manure Spill," *The State Journal-
Register*, http://www.sj-r.com/article/20111220/news/312209912 (December 20,
2011).

53. Gidon Eshel, Alon Shepon, et al., "Land, Irrigation Water, Greenhouse
Gas, and Reactive Nitrogen Burdens of Meat, Eggs, and Dairy Production in the
United States," *Proceedings of the National Academy of Sciences of the United States
of America* 111.33 (August 19, 2014).

54. David Pimentel and Marcia Pimentel," Sustainability of Meat-Based and
Plant-Based Diets and the Environment," *American Journal of Clinical Nutrition*
78 (suppl, 2003): 660S–663S, http://ajcn.nutrition.org/content/78/3/660S.full.

55. Jeremy Woods, Adrian Williams, John K. Hughes, Mairi Black, Richard
Murphy. "Energy and the Food System," *Philosophical Transactions of the Royal
Society B* 365 (August 16, 2010): 2991–3006; DOI: 10.1098/rstb.2010.0172,
http://www.ncbi.nlm.nih.gov/pmc/articles/PMC2935130/ (2016) and author
phone interview with Helen Harwatt, June 4, 2016.

56. "WHO Calls for Urgent Action to Protect Health from Climate
Change," World Health Organization, http://www.who.int/globalchange/global

-campaign/cop21/en/ (n.d.); and Linda Rudolph and Solange Gould, "Why We Need Climate, Health, and Equity in All Policies," Public Health Institute, Commentary, Institute of Medicine of the National Academies, https://cpehn .org/sites/default/files/rudolphiomclimatehealthequity.pdf (December 4, 2014).

57. P. J. Gerber, H. Steinfeld, B. Henderson, A. Mottet, C. Opio, J. Dijkman, A. Falcucci, and G. Tempio, "Tackling Climate Change through Livestock: A Global Assessment of Emissions and Mitigation Opportunities," Food and Agriculture Organization of the United Nations (FAO), Rome, http://www.fao .org/docrep/018/i3437e/i3437e.pdf (2013).

58. "Causes of Climate Change," Environmental Protection Agency, https://www3.epa.gov/climatechange/ghgemissions/gases.html (February 23 2016).

59. "Climate Change Science Overview," Environmental Protection Agency, https://www3.epa.gov/climatechange/science/overview.html (February 23, 2016).

60. P. D. Smith, et al., "Agriculture," *Climate Change 2007: Mitigation. Contribution of Working Group III to the Fourth Assessment Report of the Intergovernmental Panel on Climate Change Cambridge*, United Kingdom and New York, http://www.ipcc.ch/pdf/assessment-report/ar4/wg3/ar4_wg3_full _report.pdf (2007).

61. Bojana Bajzelj, et al., "Importance of Food-Demand Management for Climate Mitigation," *Nature*, http://www.nature.com/articles/nclimate2353 .epdf?referrer_access_token=69sDGUcUkP14CR0k0xndT9RgN0jAjWel9jnR 3ZoTv0NlteOOXpRG5bZ0W0svZ8g2c428ui7nBJcNYmaQvXtKPAPVN rdJCHVbJ8LLTz1kVuA3GfzpukWdnj5-DBmguo2z (August 31, 2014); and Rob Bailey, Antony Froggatt, and Laura Wellesley, "Livestock: Climate Change's Forgotten Sector," Royal Institute of International Affairs, http:://www.chat hamhouse.org/sites/files/chathamhouse/field/field_document/20141203 LivestockClimateChangeBaileyFroggattWellesley.pdf (December 2014).

62. Peter Scarborough, Paul N. Appleby, et al. "Dietary Greenhouse Gas Emissions of Meat-Eaters, Fish-Eaters, Vegetarians and Vegans in the UK," *Climatic Change* 125 (June 11, 2014): 179–192.

63. Bailey, Froggatt, and Wellesley, "Livestock: Climate Change's Forgotten Sector."

64. Brent Kim, Roni Neff, et al., "The Importance of Reducing Animal Product Consumption and Wasted Food in Mitigating Catastrophic Climate Change," Johns Hopkins Center for a Livable Future, http://www.jhsph.edu/ research/centers-and-institutes/johns-hopkins-center-for-a-livable-future/_pdf /research/clf_reports/2015-12-07e-role-of-diet-food-waste-in-cc-targets.pdf (December 2015).

65. Bajzelj, "Importance of Food-Demand Management for Climate Mitigation."

66. "Hampton Creek, Named by Bill Gates as One of Three Companies Shaping the Future of Food, Debuts First Product at Whole Foods Market," *Business Wire*, http://www.businesswire.com/news/home/20130920005149/en /Hampton-Creek-Named-Bill-Gates-Companies-Shaping (September 20, 2013); and India Leigh, "Are the Days Numbered for the Egg?" *Huffington Post*, http://www.huffingtonpost.co.uk/india-leigh/eggs-are-the-days-numbered_b _3327717.html (May 24, 2013).

67. Emily Cassidy, Paul West, et al., "Redefining Agricultural Yields: From Tonnes to People Nourished Per Hectare," *Environmental Research Letters* 8.3 (August 1, 2013).

68. "Food, Farming, and Hunger," Oxfam America, http://www.oxfam america.org/take-action/campaign/food-farming-and-hunger/ (2015).

69. Cassidy, West, et al., "Redefining Agricultural Yields."

70. Helen Harwatt phone interview with the author, June 4, 2016.

71. "Cholesterol Content of Foods," UCSF Medical Center, http://www .ucsfhealth.org/education/cholesterol_content_of_foods/ (n.d.).

72. "Destructive Fishing," Marine Conservation Institute, https://www .marine-conservation.org/what-we-do/program-areas/how-we-fish/destructive -fishing/ (n.d.).

73. "Responsible Fishing: Stopping Overfishing," Oceana, http://oceana.org /en/our-work/promote-responsible-fishing/bottom-trawling/learn-act/more-on -bottom-trawling-gear (n.d.).

74. Ibid.

75. "Bottom Trawls: Fishing Gear and Risks to Protected Species," National Oceanic and Atmospheric Administration, http://www.nmfs.noaa.gov/pr /interactions/gear/bottomtrawl.htm (January 30, 2014).

76. Richard Harris, "Whales, Dolphins Are Collateral Damage in Our Taste for Seafood," National Public Radio, http://www.npr.org/blogs/ thesalt/2014/01/07/260555381/thousands-of-whales-dolphins-killed-to-satisfy -our-seafood-appetite (January 8, 2014).

77. "Whaling," Whale and Dolphin Conservation, http://us.whales.org/wdc -in-action/whaling (n.d.).

78. "Overfishing: Plenty of Fish in the Sea? Not Always," *National Geographic*, http://ocean.nationalgeographic.com/ocean/critical-issues -overfishing/ (n.d.).

79. Trisha Atwood, et al., "Predators Help Protect Carbon Stocks in Blue Carbon Ecosystems," *Nature Climate Change*, https://www.researchgate.net

/publication/282327218_Predators_help_protect_carbon_stocks_in_blue
_carbon_ecosystems (September 28, 2015).

80. "An HSUS Report: The Welfare of Animals in the Aquaculture Industry,"
Humane Society of the United States, http://www.humanesociety.org/assets
/pdfs/farm/hsus-the-welfare-of-animals-in-the-aquaculture-industry-1.pdf (n.d.).

81. "Aquaculture Topics and Activities: Aquaculture," Food and Agriculture
Organization, Rome, http://www.fao.org/fishery/aquaculture/en (August 10,
2015).

82. "An HSUS Report: The Welfare of Animals in the Aquaculture
Industry"; and Stephanie Yue Cottee and Paul Petersan, "Animal Welfare and
Organic Aquaculture in Open Systems," *Journal of Agricultural and
Environmental Ethics*, http://www.humanesociety.org/assets/pdfs/farm/organic
_aquaculture.pdf (April 30, 2009).

83. "General Approach to Fish Welfare and to the Concept of Sentience
in Fish," Scientific Opinion of the Panel on Animal Health and Welfare,
http://www.efsa.europa.eu/sites/default/files/scientific_output/files/main
_documents/ahaw_op_ej954_generalfishwelfare_en.pdf (September 22, 2009).

84. Cathy Unruh, "Do Animals Have Emotions?" blog post, http://cathy
unruh.com/blog/?p=64 (n.d.).

85. "'Genius' Claim for Sticklebacks," *BBC News*, http://news.bbc.co.uk/2/hi
/uk_news/scotland/edinburgh_and_east/8104759.stm (June 17, 2009).

86. G. Bernardi, "The Use of Tools by Wrasses (Labridae)," Department
of Ecology and Evolutionary Biology, University of California Santa Cruz,
http://bio.research.ucsc.edu/people/bernardi/Bernardi/Publications/2011Tools
.pdf (2011).

87. Stephanie Yue, "An HSUS Report: The Welfare of Farmed Fish at
Slaughter," Humane Society of the United States, http://www.humanesociety
.org/assets/pdfs/farm/hsus-the-welfare-of-farmed-fish-at-slaughter.pdf (n.d.).

88. "About Fish," Compassion in World Farming, http://www.ciwf.org.uk
/farm-animals/fish/?gclid=CNmrofDwz8ICFRSGfgod0xQAbQ (2015).

89. Richard Schwartz, "Franz Kafka (1883–1924)," International Vegetarian
Union, http://www.ivu.org/history/europe20a/kafka.html (n.d.).

Chapter 4: Aligning Our Plates with Our Values

1. Ken Chadwick, phone interview with the author, June 8, 2016.

2. Roy E. Baumeister, et al., "Ego Depletion: Is the Active Self a Limited
Resource?" *Journal of Personality and Social Psychology* 74.5 (1998): 1252–1265,
http://www.psychologytoday.com/files/attachments/584/baumeisteretal1998.pdf.

3. Ibid.

4. Jonathan Haidt, *The Happiness Hypothesis: Finding Modern Truth in Ancient*

Wisdom (New York: Basic Books, 2006), http://www.happinesshypothesis.com
/happiness-hypothesis-ch1.pdf.

5. Ibid.

6. Richard H. Thaler, "Opting in vs. Opting Out," *New York Times*
http://www.nytimes.com/2009/09/27/business/economy/27view.html?_r=0
(September 26, 2009).

7. Brigitte C. Madrian and Dennis F. Shea, "The Power of Suggestion: Inertia
in 401(k) Participation and Savings Behavior," *Quarterly Journal of Economics*
116.4 (November 2001), http://www.retirementmadesimpler.org/Library
/The%20Power%20of%20Suggestion-%20Inertia%20in%20401%28k%29.pdf.

8. Milena Esherick, "Creating an Environment for Change," Whole Foods
Market, Oakland, CA (April 21, 2014).

9. Linda Lewis Griffith, "New Year's Resolutions: Why Can't We Make
Changes Stick?" *San Luis Obispo Tribune*, http://www.sanluisobispo.com
/2014/12/30/3419435/new-years-resolutions-why-cant.html (December 30,
2014).

10. Ibid.

11. "Friends and Family May Play a Role in Obesity," National Institutes of
Health, http://www.nih.gov/researchmatters/august2007/08132007obesity.htm
(August 13, 2007).

12. Amy Gorin, et al., "Involving Support Partners in Obesity Treatment,"
Journal of Consulting and Clinical Psychology 73.2 (April 2005): 341–343.

13. Loran F. Nordgren, Joop van der Pligt, and Frenk van Harreveld, "The
Instability of Health Cognitions: Visceral States Influence Self-efficacy and
Related Health Beliefs," *Journal of Health Psychology* 27.6 (2008): 722–727.

14. James E. Painter, et al., "How Visibility and Convenience Influence
Candy Consumption," University of Illinois Food and Brand Lab,
http://foodpsychology.cornell.edu/sites/default/files/candyconsumption
-2002.pdf (2002).

15. Patricia Pliner, et al., "Compliance without Pressure: Some Further Data
on the Foot-in-the-Door Technique," *Journal of Experimental Social Psychology*
10.1 (January 1974): 17–22. http://www.sciencedirect.com/science/article
/pii/0022103174900535. Accessed 5 July 2016.

16. Alice M. Tybout and Richard F. Yalch, "The Effect of Experience: A
Matter of Salience?" *Journal of Consumer Research* 6 (March 1980). http://media
.cbsm.com/uploads/1/TheEffectofExperience.pdf.

17. William R. Swinyard and Michael L. Ray, "Advertising-Selling
Interactions," Stanford School of Business, research paper no 318, http://www
.gsb.stanford.edu/faculty-research/working-papers/advertising-selling
-interactions (1976).

18. Gert Cornelissen, et al., "Positive Cueing: Promoting Sustainable Consumer Behavior by Cueing Common Environmental Behaviors as Environmental," Catholic University of Leuven, Belgium, *International Journal of Research in Marketing* 25.1 (March 2008): 46–45, https://lirias.kuleuven.be /bitstream/123456789/121057/1/MO_0.

19. Milena Esherick, personal interview with the author, May 25, 2016.

20. Natalia Angulo, "Making Meatless Mondays Stick," Fox News, http://www.foxnews.com/leisure/2013/02/04/making-meatless-mondays-stick / (February 4, 2013).

21. Sharon Palmer, "In the Studio with Peggy Neu, President of Meatless Monday," http://sharonpalmer.com/2014-10-01-in-the-studio-with-sharon -peggy-neu-president-of-meatless-monday/ (October 1, 2014).

22. Mark Bittman, "Vegan Before Six," New York: Random House (2013).

23. "The Menus of Change Initiative," Culinary Institute of America, http://www.menusofchange.org (2016).

24. Walter Willett biography, *US News & World Report*, http://www.usnews .com/topics/author/walter-c-willett-md (2016); and "Principles of Healthy, Sustainable Menus," Culinary Institute of American," http://www.menusof change.org/news-insights/resources/moc-principles/ (2016).

25. Kathryn Asher, et al., "Study of Current and Former Vegetarians and Vegans," Faunalytics, https://faunalytics. org/a-summary-of-faunalytics-study-of-current-and-former-vegetarians-and -vegans/ (December 2014).

26. Warren Ransom, "Sushi & Sashimi Information," SushiFAQ.com, http://www.sushifaq.com/sushi-sashimi-info/ (2015).

Chapter 5: So What the Heck Do I Eat?

1. Ken Botts, personal interview with the author, August 21, 2015.

2. Dan Childs, "Adios, A-Meat-Gos…Texas College Caf Goes Vegan," ABC News, http://abcnews.go.com/blogs/health/2011/09/01/adios-a-meat-gos-texas -college-caf-goes-vegan/ (September 1, 2011).

3. Bruce Horovitz, "Vegetables Shift to Center of the Plate," *USA Today*, http://www.usatoday.com/story/money/business/2013/11/09/vegetables-culinary -trends-restaurant-menus/3417879/ (November 11, 2013).

4. "Great Value Lentil, 16 oz," Walmart, http://www.walmart.com/ip/Great -Value-Lentil-16-Oz/10314942 (2016).

5. "85% Lean/ 15% Fat, Ground Beef Roll, 1 lb," Walmart, http://www .walmart.com/ip/Ground-Beef-Roll-85-Lean-1-lb/44001563 (2016).

6. Kim Willsher, "France's Top Chef Alain Ducasse Reduces amount of Meat

on the Menu," *The Guardian*. http://www.theguardian.com/lifeandstyle/2014/sep
/05/france-chef-alain-ducasse-bans-meat (September 5, 2014).

7. CookingSchools.com, "An Interview with Vegan Chef Alex Bury,"
http://cookingschools.com/resources/an-interview-with-vegan-chef-alex-bury
/#sthash.bX0N38bW.dpuf (n.d.).

8. Botts, personal interview.

9. Jane Brody, "Final Advice from Dr. Spock: Eat Only All Your Vegetables,"
New York Times, http://www.nytimes.com/1998/06/20/us/final-advice-from-dr
-spock-eat-only-all-your-vegetables.html (June 20, 1998).

10. David Linden, "Food, Pleasure and Evolution," *Psychology Today*,
https://www.psychologytoday.com/blog/the-compass-pleasure/201103/food
-pleasure-and-evolution (March 30, 2011).

11. Ibid.

12. Anthony Williams, phone interview with the author, June 10, 2016.

13. "Soyfoods Are Part of America's History," Soyfoods Association of North
America, http://www.soyfoods.org/press-releases/soyfoods-are-part-of-americas
-history (n.d.).

14. William Shurtleff and Akiko Aoyagi, "History of Meat Alternatives," Soy
Info Center, http://www.soyinfocenter.com/pdf/179/MAL.pdf (2014).

15. Michele Simon, "U.S. Meat Substitutes Market to Grow, Experts Find,"
Plant Based Foods Association, https://www.plantbasedfoods.org/u-s-meat
-substitutes-market-to-grow-experts-find/ (April 26, 2016).

16. Oscar Rousseau, "Meat Substitute Market Expected to Hit $5.2bn by
2020," *Global Meat News*, http://www.globalmeatnews.com/Analysis/Meat
-substitute-market-expected-to-hit-5.2bn-by-2020 (February 25, 2016).

17. Jonathan Kauffman, "Artisanal Vegan Cheese Comes into its Own," *San
Francisco Chronicle*, http://www.sfgate.com/food/article/Artisanal-vegan-cheese
-comes-into-its-own-6005937.php (January 12, 2015).

18. Michael Greger, "Are Fatty Foods Addictive?" NutritionFacts.org, vol. 15,
http://nutritionfacts.org/video/are-fatty-foods-addictive/# (November 20, 2013).

Chapter 6: Fill Your Plate:
Getting Protein (and Other Important Nutrients)

1. David Carter, "About David Carter," The 300 lb Vegan, http://www.the
300poundvegan.com/about-david-carter (2015).

2. Kay Lazar, "NFL Players Union and Harvard Team Up on Landmark
Study of Football Injuries and Illness," *Boston Globe*, http://www.boston.com
/lifestyle/health/2013/01/29/nfl-players-union-and-harvard-team-landmark
-study-football-injuries-and-illness/aCGnf96h7ptWX2Lnp5MIiP/story.html
(January 29, 2013).

3. Jarrett Bell, "Study Shows NFL Players Live Longer," *USA Today*, http://usatoday30.usatoday.com/sports/football/nfl/story/2012–05–08/Study-shows-NFL-players-live-longer/54847564/1 (May 8, 2012); and "NFL Mortality Study. National Institute for Occupational Safety and Health." U.S. Department of Health and Human Services http://www.cdc.gov/niosh/pdfs/nflfactsheet.pdf (January 1994).

4. David Carter, "Guest Commentary: Plant-Based Diet Leads Helps Fuel Top Performance," *Oakland Tribune*, http://www.contracostatimes.com/opinion/ci_25630071/guest-commentary-plant-based-diet-leads-helps-fuel (2014).

5. "The Compassionate Athlete: Athletes Tackle Questions about Plant Based Eating," Vegan Outreach, http://veganoutreach.org/CA.pdf (March 2015).

6. Maryann Tomovich Jacobsen, "Protein: Are You Getting Enough?" http://www.webmd.com/food-recipes/protein (2014).

7. Michael Greger, "Do Vegetarians Get Enough Protein?," Nutrition Facts, vol. 19, http://nutritionfacts.org/video/do-vegetarians-get-enough-protein/ (June 6, 2014).

8. Ibid.

9. "Protein," Harvard School of Public Health, http://www.hsph.harvard.edu/nutritionsource/what-should-you-eat/protein/ (2015).

10. Laurie Endicott Thomas, "The Myth of Protein Deficiency," Gorilla Protein, http://www.gorillaprotein.com/protein_deficiency.html (n.d.).

11. Neil Osterweil, "The Benefits of Protein," http://www.webmd.com/men/features/benefits-protein (n.d.).

12. "Protein," Harvard School of Public Health.

13. Tony C. Dreibus, "Quinoa Rides the 'Superfoods' Wave," *Wall Street Journal*, http://www.wsj.com/articles/quinoa-rides-the-superfoods-gluten-free-waves-1404926555 (July 29, 2014).

14. "Protein Foods," American Diabetes Association, http://www.diabetes.org/food-and-fitness/food/what-can-i-eat/making-healthy-food-choices/meat-and-plant-based-protein.html#sthash.ZaU6fNbF.dpuf (August 26, 2014).

15. Jacobsen, "Protein: Are You Getting Enough?"

16. "Morbidity and Mortality Weekly Report Recommendations to Prevent and Control Iron Deficiency in the United States." Centers for Disease Control and Prevention, 47(RR-3, April 3, 1998): 1–36, http://www.cdc.gov/mmwr/preview/mmwrhtml/00051880.htm.

17. Jack Norris, "Iron," Vegan Health, http://www.veganhealth.org/articles/iron (June 2013).

18. Ibid.

19. Jack Norris and Virginia Messina. *Vegan for Life: Everything You Need to Know to Be Healthy and Fit on a Plant-Based Diet.* Cambridge, MA: DaCapo Lifelong (2011).

20. "Vitamin B12 Dietary Supplement Fact Sheet," National Institutes of Health, http://ods.od.nih.gov/factsheets/VitaminB12-HealthProfessional/ (June 24, 2011).

21. Jack Norris, "Vitamin B12: Are You Getting It?" http.veganhealth.org /articles/vitaminb12 (n.d.).

22. Michael Greger, "Vegan B12 Deficiency: Putting It into Perspective," Nutrition Facts, http://nutritionfacts.org/2011/08/25/vegan-b12-deficiency -putting-it-into-perspective/ (August 25, 2011).

23. Michael Greger, "Safest Source of B12," Nutrition Facts, http://nutrition facts.org/video/safest-source-of-b12/ (February 6, 2012).

24. Michael Greger, "Cheapest Source of Vitamin B12," Nutrition Facts, http://nutritionfacts.org/video/cheapest-source-of-vitamin-b12/ (February 7, 2012).

25. Reed Mangels, "Vitamin B12 in the Vegan Diet," Vegetarian Resource Group, http://www.vrg.org/nutrition/b12.php (n.d.).

26. "Basic Report: 11164, Collards, Frozen, Chopped, Cooked, Boiled, Drained, Without Salt," USDA Nutrient List, https://ndb.nal.usda.gov/ndb /foods/show?ndbno=11164&fg=11&man=&lfacet=&format=Abridged&count &max=25&offset=0&sort=c&qlookup=&rptfrm=nl&nutrient1=301& nutrient2=&nutrient3=&subset=0&totCount=787&measureby=m (2016); and "Basic Report: 01085, Milk, nonfat, fluid, with added vitamin A and vitamin D (fat free or skim)," USDA Nutrient List, https://ndb.nal.usda.gov/ ndb/foods /show?ndbno=01085&fg=1&man=&lfacet=&format=Abridged&count=&max =25&offset=75&sort=c&qlookup =&rptfrm=nl&nutrient1=301&nutrient2 =&nutrient3=&subset=0&totCount=270&measureby=m (2016).

27. "Applying for Funding," Dairy Max, http://www.dairymax.org/apply -funding (2015); "Funding Opportunities for Your School: Earn Up to $2000* to Promote 3 Servings of Dairy Every Day!" St. Louis District Dairy Council, http://www.stldairycouncil.org/Community-Programs/Dollars-For-Dairy / (2015); "Healthy Eating Made Easier," Dairy Council of California, http://www.healthyeating.org (2015); and "Mobile Daily Classroom," Dairy Council of California, http://www.healthyeating.org/Schools/Mobile-Dairy -Classroom.aspx (2015).

28. "Top Food Sources of Saturated Fat among US Population, 2005–2006," National Cancer Institute, NHANES, http://appliedresearch.cancer.gov/diet

/foodsources/sat_fat/sf.html (October 18, 2013).

29. Susan S. Lang, "Lactose Intolerance Seems Linked to Ancestral Struggles with Harsh Climate and Cattle Diseases, Cornell Study Finds," *Cornell Chronicle*, http://www.news.cornell.edu/stories/2005/06/lactose-intolerance -linked-ancestral-struggles-climate-diseases (June 1, 2005).

30. "Milk and Dairy Allergy," American College of Allergy, Asthma & Immunology, http://acaai.org/allergies/types-allergies/food-allergy/types-food -allergy/milk-dairy-allergy (2014).

31. Caitlin Yoshiko Kandil, "5 Non-Dairy Foods With Calcium," *US News and World Report*, http://health.usnews.com/health-news/living-well-usn /articles/2012/03/14/5-non-dairy-foods-with-calcium (March 14, 2012); Michael Greger, "Plant vs. Cow Calcium," *Nutrition Facts* 2 (September 5, 2008), http://nutritionfacts.org/video/plant-vs-cow-calcium-2/; and "Appendix B: Food Sources of Selected Nutrients," Dietary Guidelines for Americans, http://www .health.gov/dietaryguidelines/dga2005/document/html/appendixb.htm (July 9, 2008).

32. Greger, Plant vs. Cow Calcium; "Dairy Cattle Management Practices in the United States, 2014," U.S. Department of Agriculture, https://www.aphis .usda.gov/animal_health/nahms/dairy/downloads/dairy14/Dairy14_dr_PartI.pdf (2014); Stacy Sneeringer, et al., "Economics of Antibiotic Use in U.S. Livestock Production," U.S. Department of Agriculture, http://www.ers.usda.gov/media /1950577/err200.pdf (November 2015); Nolan Feeney, "Illegal Antibiotics Could Be in Your Milk, FDA Finds," *Time*, http://time.com/3738069/fda-dairy -farmers-antibiotics-milk/ (March 9, 2015).

33. "Omega-3 Fatty Acids: An Essential Contribution," Harvard School of Public Health, http://www.hsph.harvard.edu/nutritionsource/omega-3/ (n.d.); and B. C. Davis and Kris-Etherton, "Achieving Optimal Essential Fatty Acid Status in Vegetarians: Current Knowledge and Practical Implications," *American Journal of Clinical Nutrition* 78 (3 Suppl, September 2003): 640S–646S, http://www.ncbi.nlm.nih.gov/pubmed/12936959.

34. "Omega-3 Fatty Acids," Harvard School of Public Health; and Jack Norris, "Omega-3 Fatty Acid Recommendations for Vegetarians," Vegan Health, http://www.veganhealth.org/articles/omega3#summ (November 2014).

35. "Omega-3 Fatty Acids," Harvard School of Public Health.

36. Michael Greger, "Hair Testing for Mercury," *Nutrition Facts*, http://nutritionfacts.org/video/hair-testing-for-mercury/ (November 30, 2010); Michael Greger, "Is Fish Oil Just Snake Oil?" *Nutrition Facts* 17 (February 3, 2014), http://nutritionfacts.org/video/is-fish-oil-just-snake-oil/; Michael Greger, "Fish and Diabetes," *Nutrition Facts* 18 (May 2), http://nutritionfacts.org /video/fish-and-diabetes; and "PCBs and Human Health," U.S. Environmental

Protection Agency, http://www.epa.gov/hudson/humanhealth.htm (2010).

37. Joel Fuhrman, "What Vegans May be Missing," https://www.drfuhrman .com/library/what_vegans_may_be_missing-DHA.aspx (n.d.); and Alison Aubrey, "Getting Brain Food Straight from the Source," National Public Radio, http://www.npr.org/templates/story/story.php?storyId=15823852 (November 1, 2007).

38. Michael Greger, "Fish Oil in Troubled Waters," *Nutrition Facts* 5 (October 5, 2011), http://nutritionfacts.org/video/fish-oil-in-troubled-waters/.

39. Peter Whoriskey, "Business Fish Oil Pills: A $1.2 Billion Industry Built, So Far, on Empty Promises," *Washington Post*, http://www.washingtonpost.com /business/economy/claims-that-fish-oil-boosts-health-linger despite science -saying-the-opposite/2015/07/08/db7567d2–1848–11e5-bd7f-4611a60dd8e5 _story.html (July 8, 2015).

40. "Omega-3 Fatty Acids," Harvard School of Public Health.

Chapter 7: Vegetable Stock:
Ingredients, Shopping, Swaps, and Other Basics

1. "Meat Substitution Tip Sheet," USA Dry Pea & Lentil Council, http://www.cookingwithpulses.com/tag/pulses-vs-meats/ (2015).

2. Jen Hathwell, "Top-10 Health Benefits of Chia Seeds," SF-Gate.com, http://healthyeating.sfgate.com/top-10-health-benefits-chia-seeds-6962.html (n.d.).

3. Elaine Magee, "The Benefits of Flaxseed," http://www.webmd.com/diet /benefits-of-flaxseed (July 20, 2011).

4. Christina Chaey, "Everything You Need to Know About How to Eat Hemp Seeds," *Bon Appetit*, http://www.bonappetit.com/test-kitchen/ingredients /article/hemp-seeds (May 11, 2015).

5. Christina Chaey, "Everything You Need to Know About Nutritional Yeast, Nature's Cheeto Dust," *Bon Appetit*, http://www.bonappetit.com/test-kitchen /ingredients/article/nutritional-yeast-2 (June 4, 2015).

METRIC CONVERSIONS

The recipes in this book have not been tested with metric measurements, so some variations might occur. Remember that the weight of dry ingredients varies according to the volume or density factor: 1 cup of flour weighs far less than 1 cup of sugar, and 1 tablespoon doesn't necessarily hold 3 teaspoons.

GENERAL FORMULA FOR METRIC CONVERSION

Ounces to grams	multiply ounces by 28.35
Grams to ounces	multiply grams by 0.035
Pounds to grams	multiply pounds by 453.5
Pounds to kilograms	multiply pounds by 0.45
Cups to liters	multiply cups by 0.24
Fahrenheit to Celsius	subtract 32 from Fahrenheit temperature, multiply by 5, divide by 9
Celsius to Fahrenheit	multiply Celsius temperature by 9, divide by 5, add 32

VOLUME (LIQUID) MEASUREMENTS

1 teaspoon	= ⅙ fluid ounce	= 5 milliliters
1 tablespoon	= ½ fluid ounce	= 15 milliliters
2 tablespoons	= 1 fluid ounce	= 30 milliliters
¼ cup	= 2 fluid ounces	= 60 milliliters
⅓ cup	= 2⅔ fluid ounces	= 79 milliliters
½ cup	= 4 fluid ounces	= 118 milliliters
1 cup or ½ pint	= 8 fluid ounces	= 250 milliliters
2 cups or 1 pint	= 16 fluid ounces	= 500 milliliters
4 cups or 1 quar	= 32 fluid ounces	= 1,000 milliliters
1 gallon	= 4 liters	

WEIGHT (MASS) MEASUREMENTS

1 ounce	= 30 grams	
2 ounces	= 55 grams	
3 ounces	= 85 grams	
4 ounces	= ¼ pound	= 125 grams
8 ounces	= ½ pound	= 240 grams
12 ounces	= ¾ pound	= 375 grams
16 ounces	= 1 pound	= 454 grams

OVEN TEMPERATURE EQUIVALENTS, FAHRENHEIT (F) AND CELSIUS (C)

100°F	= 38°C
200°F	= 95°C
250°F	= 120°C
300°F	= 150°C
350°F	= 180°C
400°F	= 205°C
450°F	= 230°C

VOLUME (DRY) MEASUREMENTS

¼ teaspoon	= 1 milliliter
½ teaspoon	= 2 milliliters
¾ teaspoon	= 4 milliliters
1 teaspoon	= 5 milliliters
1 tablespoon	= 15 milliliters
¼ cup	= 59 milliliters
⅓ cup	= 79 milliliters
½ cup	= 118 milliliters
⅔ cup	= 158 milliliters
¾ cup	= 177 milliliters
1 cup	= 225 milliliters
4 cups or 1 quart	= 1 liter
½ gallon	= 2 liters
1 gallon	= 4 liters

LINEAR MEASUREMENTS

½ inch	= 1½ cm
1 inch	= 2½ cm
6 inches	= 15 cm
8 inches	= 20 cm
10 inches	= 25 cm
12 inches	= 30 cm
20 inches	= 50 cm

Resources

Recommended Reading

Cooking

Isa Does It: Amazingly Easy, Wildly Delicious Vegan Recipes for Every Day of the Week, by Isa Chandra Moskowitz (New York: Little, Brown and Co., 2013).

Vegan With a Vengeance, by Isa Chandra Moskowitz (Boston, MA: Da Capo Lifelong, 2015).

The Vegan Table: 200 Unforgettable Recipes for Entertaining Every Guest at Every Occasion, by Colleen Patrick-Goudreau (Beverly, MA: Fair Winds Press, 2009).

Vegan on the Cheap, by Robin Robertson (New York: Houghton Mifflin Harcourt, 2010).

Crossroads: Extraordinary Recipes from the Restaurant That Is Reinventing Vegan Cuisine, by Tal Ronnen (Sioux City, IA: Artisan Press, 2015).

The Homemade Vegan Pantry: The Art of Making Your Own Staples, by Miyoko Schinner (Berkeley, CA: Ten Speed Press, 2015).

Health and Lifestyle

The Get Healthy, Go Vegan Cookbook: 125 Easy and Delicious Recipes to Jump-Start Weight Loss and Help You Feel Great, by Neal Barnard, MD (Boston, MA: Da Capo Lifelong, 2010).

Living the Farm Sanctuary Life: The Ultimate Guide to Eating Mindfully, Living Longer, and Feeling Better Every Day, by Gene Baur and Gene Stone (Emmaus, PA: Rodale Books, 2015)

Veganist: Lose Weight, Get Healthy, Change the World, by Kathy Freston (New York: Weinstein Books, 2011).

Eat to Live, by Joel Fuhrman, MD (New York: Little, Brown and Co., 2011).

How Not to Die, by Michael Greger, MD (Charleston, SC: CreateSpace, 2016).

The Complete Idiot's Guide to Plant-Based Nutrition, by Julieanna Hever, RD (Orlando, FL: Alpha Press, 2011).

Vegan for Life, by Jack Norris, RD and Virginia Messina, MPH, RD (Boston, MA: Da Capo Lifelong, 2011).

The 30-Day Vegan Challenge, by Colleen Patrick-Goudreau (Montali Press, 2015).

Animals

Second Nature: The Inner Lives of Animals, by Jonathan Balcombe (New York: Palgrave Macmillan, 2010).

Farm Sanctuary: Changing Hearts and Minds About Animals and Food, by Gene Baur (New York: Touchstone, 2008).

Farmageddon: The True Cost of Cheap Meat, by Philip Lymbery (New York: Bloomsbury, 2014).

The Humane Economy, by Wayne Pacelle (New York: William Morrow, 2016).

Eating Animals, by Jonathan Safran Foer (Boston: Back Bay Books, 2010).

Dominion: The Power of Man, the Suffering of Animals, and the Call to Mercy, by Matthew Scully (New York: St. Martin's Griffin, 2003).

Animal Liberation, by Peter Singer (New York: Harper Perennial, 2009).

Do Unto Animals: A Friendly Guide to How Animals Live, and How We Can Make Their Lives Better, by Tracey Stewart (Sioux City, IA: Artisan Press, 2015).

Websites

Recipes

HappyHerbivore.com
HumaneSociety.org/recipes
Lighter.World
MeatlessMonday.com
MinimalistBaker.com
OlivesforDinner.com
WickedHealthyFood.com

Lifestyle

ForksOverKnives.com
HappyCow.net
JoyfulVegan.com
The30DayVeganChallenge.com
WorldofVegan.com
VegNews.com

Health

DrFuhrman.com
JackNorrisRD.com
NutritionFacts.org
VeganHealth.org

Animals

ChooseVeg.com
HumaneSociety.org
TryVeg.com

Films

Cowspiracy
Earthlings
Forks Over Knives
Vegucated

Acknowledgments

The adage attributed to Confucius, "Choose a job you love, and you will never have to work a day in your life," is mostly true. While I'd never say writing a book isn't hard work, I feel extremely fortunate to be in the position to do so. Even more, I'm humbled and honored every day to be able to work alongside some of the most intelligent, passionate, and compassionate people out there to create a more humane society for animals and people alike.

My most sincere gratitude to Ken Botts, Ken Chadwick, Isabelle Cnudde, David Carter, Helen Harwatt, Eric O'Grey, Ben Peterson, and Anthony Williams for sharing their inspiring stories. I'm indebted to Matt Prescott, Paul Shapiro, Josh Balk, Karla Dumas, Lauren Pitts, and Ashley Rhinehart for their help with edits and research, and I thank all of my HSUS Farm Animal Protection family for their ongoing support and hard work for animals.

Milena Esherick and Alex Bury, deepest thanks for the many hours of advocacy we spent together, which inspired this project—for the recipes, research support, and your friendship.

Jennifer Thompson, my wonderful sister, not only ruined eggs for me—which is a good thing—but also has always pushed me to step outside of my comfort zone and cheered me on all the while. My parents, Clyde and Sandra Sigmon, told me I could do anything I put my mind to. Words can't adequately express my gratitude for their love and support. I wrote like a MF, motivated by RaeLeann Smith, who I thank for the encouragement, love, and wisdom.

My agent Roger Freet believed in this project and has been an immense pleasure to work with. I see many more carrot dogs in our future. My editor Renee Sedliar could polish any rock into a diamond. I'm so grateful to Renee for her support of this venture as well as Da Capo publisher John Radziewicz, marketing director Kevin Hanover, publicity director Lissa Warren, and publicist Mike Giarratano.

To all the advocates working hard for animals every day, you are my heroes and I thank you from the bottom of my heart.

This project wouldn't have come to fruition without the ongoing support, encouragement, and love of my husband and partner in fighting for animals, Mark Middleton. Life with you, Calvin, Dracula, Reggie, Sebastian, and Uma gets better every day. Until every cage is empty.

Index

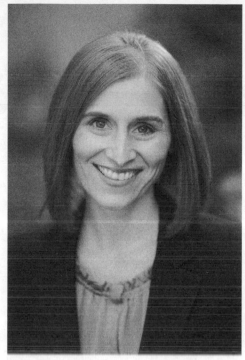

MICHELLE CEHN

About the Author

Kristie Middleton is the senior director of food policy for the Humane Society of the United States (HSUS) and a leading figure in the movement to reform our global food system. She's a sought-after speaker and thought leader on the topic. Middleton's work has been covered by national media, including the *New York Times*, the *Los Angeles Times*, Politico, CNN, and countless others.

Middleton directs the HSUS's efforts to increase plant-based eating. She's partnered with some of the nation's biggest school districts—including Los Angeles Unified, Detroit Public Schools, and Boston Public Schools—to implement Meatless Monday. And she's helped some of America's top universities develop and implement programs to add more plant-based options to their menus and train culinary staff in plant-based food prep.

Middleton holds a certificate in plant-based nutrition from T. Colin Campbell Center for Nutrition Studies. She lives with her husband, dog, and four cats in Oakland, California.